QIGONG
BASICS

QIGONG
BASICS

Paul Eng

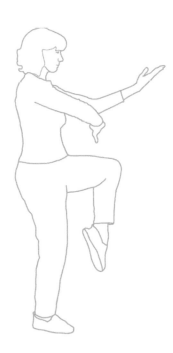

TUTTLE Publishing

Tokyo | Rutland, Vermont | Singapore

Published in 2004 by Tuttle Publishing, an imprint of Periplus Editions (HK) Ltd.
Copyright © 2004 Periplus Editions (HK) Ltd.

Library of Congress Cataloging-in-Publication Data
Elinwood, Ellae.
  Qigong basics / Ellae Elinwood.— 1st ed.
    p. cm.
  Includes bibliographical references.
  1. Qi gong. I. Title.   RA781.8.E43 2004
  613.7'148—dc22

                    2004007208

ISBN-13: 978-0-8048-4758-2

(Previously published under ISBN 978-0-8048-3585-5)

Distributed by:
North America, Latin America,
and Europe
Tuttle Publishing
364 Innovation Drive
North Clarendon, VT 05759-9436
Tel: (802) 773-8930;Fax: (802) 773-6993
info@tuttlepublishing.com
www.tuttlepublishing.com

Japan
Tuttle Publishing
Yaekari Building, 3rd Floor
5-4-12 O–saki, Shinagawa-ku
Tokyo 141-0032
Tel: (03) 5437-0171;Fax: (03) 5437-0755
sales@tuttle.co.jp
www.tuttle.co.jp

Asia Pacific
Berkeley Books Pte. Ltd.
61 Tai Seng Avenue #02-12
Singapore 534167
Tel: (65) 6280-3320; Fax: (65) 6280-6290
inquiries@periplus.com.sg
www.periplus.com.sg

First edition
22 21 20 19 18   8 7 6 5 4 3 2 1

Printed in China   1808RR

TUTTLE PUBLISHING® is a registered trade-mark of Tuttle Publishing, a division of Periplus Editions (HK) Ltd.

table of contents

Part 4: *Qigong Sequences*   107

Part 5: *Deepening Your Practice*   143

I N ORDER TO GRASP the vital necessity of qigong, one must understand qi—the force of life and the storehouse of vitality. Human beings are filled with life by qi. The amount of qi, the balance of qi, and the reservoirs of qi coursing throughout the body determine the amount of vitality, health, and inner well-being of every person. More qi, more vitality. The more balanced qi is, the more endurance and health one has. More qi awareness means more emotional well-being and spiritual development. Qigong's reason for existence is to give each practitioner a reliable, consistent, and continuously effective tool to create the best possible relationship to qi and all that qi offers.

Gong is the Chinese word used to describe the positive results of perseverance. *Qigong*, then, means benefiting from developing the continuing life energy, through perseverance. The direct benefit of practicing qigong is improved health and well-being.

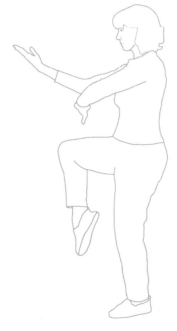

The ancient exercises of qigong were crafted to access and optimize qi and the *dan tian*—the storage vessel in the body for qi. Qigong teaches you how to take the greatest possible advantage of qi and its gifts.

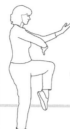

chapter 1

the history of qigong

EVERY CULTURE has a name for the energy that animates all life—qi, *chi*, bio-energy, *prana*, spirit. Qigong has the rare ability to include everyone in its experience and to adapt to the needs of many different groups without losing its own character in the process. Self-healing disciplines, spiritual renewal groups, martial arts, medicine, Buddhism, and Taoism have all incorporated aspects of qigong and benefited from its gifts. It has been incorporated into virtually every aspect of Chinese life throughout history—medicine, the arts, theater, martial arts, religion, and shamanic rituals.

The qigong practiced in the West is the result of many thousands of years of evolution. Qigong developed as China developed and has been inextricably woven into the history of the Chinese people, their society, and their culture. Qigong's influence on Chinese philosophy and the Chinese way of life has been unparalleled in its value and significance. Like a golden thread, it has been woven into so many aspects of Chinese culture that any one single beginning is impossible to trace.

Thus, the history of qigong is vague, but it does fall into several developmental phases. This chapter will explore what is known of qigong's past.

Qigong has been known by a series of names, and the name "qigong" itself is relatively recent. An ancient name was *dao yin*, which means to guide chi with intent as the arms and legs are moved and stretched. In the twentieth century, the name evolved from *chi kung* or *chi gong. Chi* is the word for "energy." *Kung* and *gong* mean "force."

The accurate pronunciation is *key gong.* You can approximate the Chinese pronunciation by running the words together. Lift the base of the tongue to the back of the throat as you say the "ng" at the end of "gong." That oral action drops the voice, giving "qi" the emphasis.

Qigong Emerges

The earliest qigong was known by many typically descriptive phrases, such as "draw in the new, dispense with the old," "moving qi," "nourishing life," and "directing or guiding qi."

The Falun Gong Society, which bases much of its training on qigong, believes that qigong's roots are prehistoric. Early human beings had a natural desire to strengthen their bodies and attune their senses and intuition to the wild natural world around them, in order to heighten their ability to survive. Prehistoric human beings were concerned with carving a life out of the seeming chaos of nature. They sought an order or pattern in nature's vast and often threatening activity, so as to find their own place in that pattern. Living in harmony with this natural order could make the life of the individual and the community more secure, prosperous, and congenial.

By practicing these principles, with the understanding that they were thus creating a connection to all of nature, these ancient people established certain basic rules and patterns to follow. The life force was perceived to include three qualities:

Heaven — *tian*
Earth — *di*
Humanity — *ren*

The three formed a natural triune and were called *San Cai*, the "Three Natural Powers." Each aspect of this natural triune—heaven, earth, and humanity—is affected by certain rules and cycles. The rules are fixed and never change. For instance, heaven, or the universe, contains the earth, and the earth contains humankind. The cycles are shifts that have a consistent, recurring pattern. For example, the earth moves in relation to the universe in a cycle. That the earth is part of the universe is a rule. As a result, seasons occur on the earth in consistent cycles. Human beings are endlessly engaged in understanding and adapting to the seasons. The cycles alter, but in a predictable pattern. The purpose of life in ancient China became the quest to live in harmony with these rules and cycles. Being successful at this improved one's ability to survive, first of all, and then improved one's quality of life. Because qigong deepens one's connection with self and omnipresent nature, it was the perfect tool

Various Spellings of Qigong

Chi Kung

Chi Gong

Tajiquan

Qigong

for increasing one's understanding of the rules and cycles and, most essentially, the role of humankind in these unending patterns.

Around 2400 B.C., the information gained from qigong and a variety of other wisdoms led to the writing of the Chinese classic *The Book of Changes*, or the *I Ching*. The *I Ching* had a profound cultural significance in the evolution of ancient China, and its enigmatic wisdom still has much to offer any reader. How does the *I Ching* pertain to qigong? In Chinese philosophy, all things are related. One thing influences another. It is not possible to understand qigong without understanding where it fits within the wholeness of life.

The *I Ching* explained the rules and cycles of life, offering both practical wisdom and spiritual nourishment. Its wisdom encompassed the natural rhythms of seasons, weather, climate, changes of rain, heat, cold, and drought. It taught that these earth cycles were born from the heavenly cycles of day and night, months and years. Natural rules and cycles, the obvious and the subtle, were arrangements of the San Cai.

Practicing qigong and studying the *I Ching* confer an understanding of the web that humanity is woven into, of the rules and cycles that govern human life. This understanding facilitates correct timing in action or non-action—and it is this ability to interact harmoniously with the natural order that determines the success of an individual, community, or nation. Hunting, planting, communication, action or non-action, situating and building a home, birth control, the arrangement of elements to enhance vitality (*feng shui*), political trends, floods, famines, birth, and death are all made easier by appropriate timing — or

I Ching

*C*arl Jung, the Swiss psychologist, was fascinated with the enigmatic and highly accurate wisdom of the I Ching. In writing the foreword for the Western translation in 1949, he wrote: "The manner in which the I Ching tends to look upon reality seems to disfavor our causative procedures. The moment under actual observation appears to the ancient Chinese view more of a chance hit than a clearly defined result of concurring causal chain processes. The matter of interest seems to be the configuration formed by chance events in the moment of observation, and not at all the hypothetical reasons that seemingly account for the coincidence. While the Western mind carefully sifts, weighs, selects, classifies, isolates, the Chinese picture of the moment encompasses everything down to the minutest nonsensical detail, because all of the ingredients make up the observed moment."

harder by incorrect timing. Qi, or energy, is the definer, interpreter, and director of events, both in personal life and in nature. Not only do the San Cai, or the Three Natural Powers, influence all of life's events, but they determine them.

Living deeply embedded in nature, the ancient Chinese had no desire to challenge the San Cai.

> **Ancient Chinese Authors and Their Works on Qigong**
>
> Cao, Yuan-Bai. *Bao Shen Mi Yao*, or *The Secret Important Document of Body Protection*. 1600s.
>
> Ge Hong, *Bao Pa Zi* (*Healing the Body*).
>
> Bian Que, *Nan Jing* (*Classical Disorders*).
>
> Chen-Ji-Ru, *Yang Shen Fu Yu* (*Brief Introduction to Nourishing the Body*).

Their lives worked much better for them if they recognized their place in the San Cai and made every effort to live the dao—the natural way of life.

The Practice of Qigong for Health

The commitment to consistent and daily practice of qigong aligns the practitioner with every cycle of change, according to unalterable rules—an essential tool for interfacing harmoniously with events as they occur. The early Chinese culture achieved greater security through diligent application of dao, and in time the pressure to ensure survival became less intense for some. The knowledge of the San Cai and the commitment to living in the dao expanded. The quest to uncover the body's own natural rules and cycles began. Through the pursuit of this knowledge, the art of Chinese medicine took its first steps.

What is now the highly skilled and complex art of acupuncture has its roots in this time. The Shang dynasty (1766–1154 b.c.) provided the cultural support for the initial study of qi and its courses through the body. The first tools of acupuncture were probes made from stones. These were inserted into the body at precise points to adjust, balance, and harmonize the qi flows. This adjustment would then create a smoother alignment of the body's qi with all of nature. What doctors did with probes, qigong accomplished through breath and coordinated movements. As both methods were pursued and practiced, each deepened and expanded the effectiveness of the other.

The Zhou dynasty (1050–256 B.C.) brought forward the important link of breath, qi, and the cultivation of qi. Breath techniques were recorded and passed throughout the country. This initiated a steady stream of descriptions of breath techniques, discussions of their effectiveness, and elaborations on various qigong methods. The variety proliferated, but the common thread remained—breath and movement coordinated to achieve health and well-being through understanding the San Cai and living the dao.

*B*y the Zhou dynasty (1050–256 b.c.) the movements had continued their primitive expression by being absorbed into the rites and ceremonies of the shamans of the day. Covered with ani-mal skins, they would dance and move throughout the ritual of celebration, using qigong movements to enhance their feeling of unity with the greater power and imbuing the crowd with a "contact high," or personal experience. The bridge from early human beings to recorded history is reflected in qigong through the use of animal sounds and movements.

Qigong in Spiritual Practice

Buddhism made its way into China during the Han dynasty (206 B.C.–A.D. 220). It joined with the San Cai, and the merging created a wonderful and prosperous time for China. China's Emperor Han converted to Buddhism and incorporated the Buddha's principles of compassion and equanimity into the duties of rulership. These concepts of leadership translated into fair and just treatment for the people of China. The equanimity demonstrated by the authorities inspired the people to know Buddhism, with the result that Buddhism gained great popularity and grew rapidly into a vast religious movement. Buddhist monasteries sprang up around the country. The monk's training to walk the path toward enlightenment became a sought-after lifestyle. Qigong's ability to align with qi, balance qi, and join with all-encompassing nature became a golden tool in the monks' enlightened quest.

Qigong and meditation techniques had been used in India, where Buddha lived and taught. These Indian versions were later integrated into the Chinese-influenced Buddhist rituals and meditations. Each of the temples mushrooming throughout the country during this bountiful era taught intricate qigong/ meditation techniques. As is human, competition to be the most enlightened emerged. A variety of qigong/meditation techniques became

Qigong's ability to connect with the universal guaranteed its use in a variety of arenas and events. The events were designed to lift the weight of existence and celebrate the continuity of life. Pushing this connection to life's essence to the extreme, Wan Zi-Qiao (550 B.C.) practiced the crane dance, a form of qigong, in an attempt to arrive at immortality. He did die, nonetheless, but his followers reported that it was an unusual death. He flew away on the back of a crane. The crane dance's ability to connect with eternity was used by King Wu (514–495 B.C.) specifically to uplift him from his grief over the death of his daughter. Turning toward the divine for solace, he demanded a public demonstration of qigong's crane dance. The dance was presented as the spiritual triumph over death.

essential for the pursuit of enlightenment. Concealment was a way of life in ancient China, and it also permeated the Buddhist monasteries. The practices of self-healing, meditation, and chi sensitivity were honed for effectiveness through the dedicated attentiveness of the monks. As qigong practices increased in value and each monastery developed its own rituals, the monks became secretive about them. The hidden practices were taught verbally, in guarded, private circumstances.

India and China have shared a common border for thousands of years. India's yoga, a series of stationary postures done usually in a predictable sequence, predates qigong. Yoga bears much common ground with qigong and may have been an inspiration for the way qigong's moving postures flow in a predictable sequence.

The qigong of the lay people continued to grow, unaffected by this secret spiritual branch. Qigong as a path to enlightenment disappeared into the enigmatic world of monastic rituals, and the practice of concealing this spiritual aspect of qigong went on for centuries. The gap widened between the spiritually developed Buddhist monks and the lay people, who were seeking only health and harmony. Thus, two different forms of qigong emerged.

As the monks hid their form of qigong, the medical scholars of the day became more and more interested in the medical and philosophical potential of qigong. This exploration of qigong as a medical resource kept the practice alive in the lay culture of China. Buddhism only added intricacy to the forms

Medical doctors had a great effect on the evolution of qigong throughout the population of China (A.D. 200–400). The very famous and still revered Hua Tuo initiated the use of acupuncture (done then with stone needles) to suppress pain; Ge Hong recorded the possibilities of using the mind to guide and develop the growth of chi in the body; Tao Hong-Jin is generally credited with the first comprehensive compilation of qigong techniques.

and practices. The forms studied by medical scholars and practiced by lay people were not only far more accessible, but also easier to learn. Qigong continued to maintain its core basic value as these three different forms were absorbed and developed.

Qigong in the Martial Arts

The monasteries continued in their secret practices but reached a point where the constant repetition of the practices was causing qigong to lose its effectiveness. Enter the Indian Da Mo, who was invited by the emperor Wu of the Liang dynasty (A.D. 500–557) to teach in the royal court. He did not please the emperor and left to join a monastery. After almost a decade of meditation and reflection on the weakened condition of the monks, he taught them enhanced qigong forms to improve their health and strength. They changed from a weakened group of men, inclined to become lost in meditation, to a vibrant group of physically powerful men. The martial arts became very much a part of monastic life. Qigong improved strength and endurance so profoundly that the techniques devised by Da Mo revitalized the martial arts, and monk/ warriors were

Qigong was enhanced and taught during the Tang dynasty (A.D. 618–906) in ways that remain valuable.
In his book *Zhu Bing Yuan Hou Lu* (*A Treatise on the Origins and Symptoms of Various Diseases*), Yun Fang Chao compiled over 250 variations of the form specifically designed to improve the internal flow of qi. Si-Miao Sun developed a six-sound technique used by the Buddhists to govern the qi flows. Lao Zi introduced the concept of qi enhancement through massage. He suggested forty-nine touch techniques.

the outcome—men who sought a balance between the meditative state (yin without and yang within) and the martial state (yin within and yang without).

As the monk/warriors renewed themselves, qigong continued to develop among lay people as it was honed by a variety of doctors and scholars. This became a time of wonderfully creative approaches to qigong. The forms varied, but techniques for the improvement of health and spirit were integrated into the practice. Qigong became more encompassing. During the Song dynasty (A.D. 960–1279), the famous Shaolin temple—haven to the monk/warriors of old China—began to seriously incorporate qigong into their martial arts discipline. It is during this period that Zhang San Feng is credited with creating the t'ai chi ch'uan, or taijiquan, approach to martial arts.

Just as qigong took inspiration from the movements of animals for the Five Animal Sport form (Hua Tuo), Zhang San Feng took to heart and hand the movements he witnessed in a fight to the death between a bird (perhaps a crane) and a snake. The jumping and quick-pecking bird was soon worn down by the patient dodging of the gracefully swaying snake, until the bird was weary and the snake struck with one deadly motion. Zhang San Feng became a man inspired, and the martial arts reached a turning point. Grace, power, and refined use of raw energy became the essence of the craft.

In the second century A.D., the well-known and respected Chinese physician Hua Tuo furthered qigong's steadily evolving practices by developing therapeutic qigong exercises based on the movements of five different types of animals. The Bear, Coiling Snake, and Turning Tiger are a few. These reflections of animal grace in the practice of qigong add to the advancement of skill and to the feeling of connectedness with nature that qigong brings.

A New Era

From A.D. 1000 until 1911 there was an absolute flowering of qigong, acupressure, and acupuncture. Dr. Wang Wei-Yi provided a clear and concise illustration of the twelve qi meridians—the energy pathways—in the body. During this time a greater variety of forms (sets of exercises) was developed. Each form focused on achieving a particular goal through qi guidance and enhancement.

T'ai chi ch'uan developed initially as an interesting branch of qigong. Just as it incorporated other aspects of the Chinese culture, t'ai chi ch'uan used the flowing movements of qigong to enhance the martial artist's inner world of peaceful quiet in the violent, fast-moving action of t'ai chi ch'uan.

Although, like much of ancient Chinese history, the story may be part lore, the sage-warrior generally credited with introducing the flowing movements of nature into t'ai chi ch'uan is Zhang San Feng. One day he was observing a battle to the death between a bird and a snake. The bird would focus and attack, using beak, wings, and feet. The snake would sway and gracefully avoid contact until the bird tired. It was then the snake struck once. Once was enough. The bird was dead and the snake left the scene, still undulating gracefully. What Zhang San Feng witnessed in the bird's formidable opponent was a style of martial art that inspired him for the rest of his life. He returned to his monastery and began the integration of the grace of qigong into the heretofore fast and frequent movements of the martial arts.

The combination of motions and poses that made up these practices served to increase the strength and endurance of soldiers, to provide a wiser path to enlightenment, and to improve the overall health of the Chinese people. All of these advances made qigong more and more popular throughout China.

Qigong has entered the Western world, the distinctions between t'ai chi (not t'ai chi ch'uan) and qigong are clear. Their roots are now actually quite different. T'ai chi evolved from t'ai chi ch'uan, a martial art, and it retains these moves. Qigong is rooted in self-healing and gently extending into wholeness to find the source of ever-renewable vitality.

Before 1911 China was, for the most part, a closed, isolated society. After 1911, with the fusion of East and West, the outlying countries developed an interest in qigong, and the practices expanded. This was a time that heralded a new Chinese era. Other countries discovered the ancient holistic science practiced in China, which considered the body as a whole and made use of its natural longing to move toward health. This respect for life and the body stirred great interest in the West. Slowly China opened, bit by bit, and the world absorbed more and more of its cultural wealth and wisdom.

Qigong Today

The final stage of qigong's history is the era we are part of now. In 1973 President Richard Nixon visited China and broke the bonds of silence and concealment. As business and tourism moved back and forth between East and West, qigong's wisdom took hold. More and more people worldwide are discovering for themselves the remarkable gifts of qigong practice. In a single qigong exercise, you can reap the benefits of centuries of devoted, careful attention to honing forms to their greatest effectiveness.

Qigong was a central resource in the historical evolution of China. It was central because it provided secure access to Wu Chi—the great potential—and it further allowed effective dispersal of qi's vitality through the body. The beneficial effects of qi dispersal contributed greatly to the wisdom of Chinese medicine. This wisdom acknowledges that first and foremost all is wholeness, and that the quality of one's health and well-being results from the ability to connect, balance, and nourish one's relationship to wholeness, or dao. Qigong's nature metaphors expressed and enhanced its connectedness to everything. The awareness of connection beyond the boundaries of the body's five senses, combined with mimicking a creature's graceful movements, gave qigong practitioners the maximum advantage.

Qigong History at a Glance

2400 B.C.

Qigong emerges in China and contributes to the writing of *Yi Jing*, or *I Ching*.

Shang Dynasty (1766–1154 B.C.)

Royals, daoist monks, scholars, and lay people all practice qigong for health, well-being, and spiritual nourishment.

Stone probes were first used to affect qi flows in the body.

Zhou Dynasty (1050–256 B.C.)

The refining of breath and movement, coordinated with qi storage and refinement, is incorporated into the qigong practices.

Han Dynasty (206 b.c.–A.D. 220)

Buddhism expands throughout China and incorporates and hones qigong to enhance the path of attaining Buddhahood. This, in turn, creates an expansion of qigong into Buddhism beyond China's borders. Indian Buddhism, Daoist Buddhism, and Tibetan Buddhism all take in qigong and create their own sequences. Religious qigong develops. Qigong becomes concealed in the monasteries.

Circulation of qi is reflected upon, described, and debated among scholars and doctors in texts that are still read and remain influential.

Liang Dynasty (A.D. 500–557)

Qigong is brought into the martial arts temples. The martial arts build on intricate Buddhist practices to create an effective tool for increasing internal force.

Qigong for health and medicine continues to be practiced among the lay people.

Song Dynasty (A.D. 960–1279)

Martial artists continue their own refinement of qigong and t'ai chi as disciplines for inner and outer force. During this time many qigong styles and forms are developed and specialized.

The Modern Era

The Qing dynasty is overthrown in 1911, heralding the end of Chinese isolation and the beginning of openness to the rest of the world.

In 1973 President Richard Nixon opens China to the Western world, and qigong begins its Western expansion.

Hua Tuo represented the Chinese medical philosophy that the doctor's job was to keep the patient healthy, seeking continuously to avert illness. The patients' role was to take responsibility for their own health, using the doctor's wisdom as a guide. Patients concerned themselves with effective self-care, self-maintenance, and self-healing techniques. This concept of Chinese medicine is one of the cornerstones of the classic text *The Yellow Emperor's Classic of Internal Medicine*. Unlike Western medicine, which excels at diagnosis once a disease has taken hold, the Chinese medicine of Hua Tuo and later the *Yellow Emperor's Classic* outline methods that sensitize one to one's own healthy state. Thus, when that state begins to slip into disease, the individual and the doctor can use medical skills, intuition, and time-tested Chinese techniques to diagnose the change in the qi levels. This change or stagnation in the qi levels is the first serious step toward declining health and well-being. Once the imbalance is diagnosed, clear and concise steps can be taken to correct the imbalance and restore ease to the body, mind, and spirit.

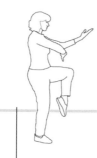

chapter 2

the philosophy
of qigong

THE CHINESE EXPLORATION of the rules, cycles, and patterns of qi has given the world an effective understanding of how to reduce inner stress. The practice of qigong has created a philosophy of cooperation with nature through the understanding and skillful guiding of three types of qi: *tian qi*, or "heaven qi"; *di qi*, or "Earth qi"; and *ren qi*, or "human qi."

Tian qi is the flow and force of the heavens, which constantly flow to the earth.

Di qi is receptive and absorbing of tian qi, which influences and changes it. This interaction is one of rebalancing to attain equilibrium, however briefly. It is this rebalancing that accounts for all the changes and challenges of climate. Di qi is a force-field pattern of qi flow lines and the earth's magnetic field. The flows and forces surround and permeate the earth.

There are various types and patterns of qi:

Breath qi: Qi internalized through taking in air/oxygen (the body separates the new qi, stores it, and releases old qi on the exhale)

Food qi: Absorbed from a live and vital food source (the importance of which cannot be overemphasized)

Genetic qi: The level of qi you have as an inheritance from your family

Internal qi: The flows inside the body

External qi: All energy extending from the body

Nurturing qi: Inside the meridians

Protecting qi: Erects a barrier of protection

Di qi flows like a force of water, moving easily here, flooding there, creating stagnation somewhere else. Its state of fluidity depends on interactions between people and the earth. Di qi has been skillfully explored and explained in the ancient art of feng shui, the art of placement.

Ren qi lives within this latticework of force fields. Ren qi is itself a personal force-field latticework, influenced in the rebalancing process by all the encompassing, constantly changing forces of di qi and tian qi. All human events, from the magnificent to the minute, from the creative to the destructive, are controlled by the interactive relationship of tian qi and di qi. It is the rule of life for human beings to live within the fabric of these interfacing forces. That can never change.

Qi functions within rules and cycles. These rules are never-changing and must be accepted; their parameters cannot be violated. Tian qi's rules govern sunshine, moonlight, the tides, and the like. Di qi's rules govern gravity, rotation, poles, and so on. Tian qi and di qi have cycles, repeated variations within the rules—varying lengths of day and night, changes in the tides, and fluctuations in the duration and intensity of the seasons. When di qi is balanced, animals and plants grow and thrive. When it is imbalanced, climatic challenges such as natural disasters occur, and all of natural life suffers. Since human beings are intricately woven by ren qi into this universal web, it is essential for us to understand that the rules are fixed and the cycles are changeable—and we must learn to adjust to these forces. It is successful adjustment that leads to a long and healthy life.

Qigong practice has been valued over the centuries and passed along because of its effectiveness in preventing illness evoked by changes in weather. It increases the internal qi, strengthens the organs, promotes better general health, and—even more exciting—extends life by blessing it with health and

Descriptive words for the force of life itself and our connection to omnipresent nature are found in every language and culture.

Ruach Ha Kodesh (Hebrew): Breath of God

Spiritus Sanctus (Latin): Holy spirit

Nafas Ruh (Islam): Soul breath

Pneuma (Greek): Vital breath

Num (African): Life energy

Nilch'i (Navajo): Life-giving wind

Ni (Lakota Sioux): Life-giving force

Ha (Hawaiian): Sacred healing breath

Chindi (Navajo): Life force

Bioenergy (Western): Life energy

Prana (Indian): Eternal elixir

Meditation

At around 3:00 a.m., qi is in the process of changing its "frequencies" from the previous day to be ready for the next day, and many meditation practitioners consider this to be a perfect time to meditate—the elixir hours, time of a soft, new day and fresh new qi.

The solid root of qigong has grown into five strong branches:

Health maintenance

Recovery from disease

Lengthening life

Martial arts

The path to enlightenment

well-being. Qigong shows the way to the source of life and well-being: qi. When ren qi is in harmonious alignment with di qi and tian qi, life is complete, balanced, and exactly as it should be.

The wholeness this harmony reveals is called dao—the complete whole. Dao is nourished by Wu Chi, the great void from which all qi—tian, di, and ren—and all else flow. As the qi flows from tian qi to di qi and ren qi, it divides into the two forces of life as we know them: yin, the feminine flow, and yang, the masculine flow. The interaction of these forces within all qi offers the opportunity for achieving creative balance. Qigong provides a simple route to balancing yin and yang. (You can strive to understand exactly what is happening as you practice qigong, or you can just let the qi do its thing and feel better afterward.)

Yin and yang join to create ren qi and flow through the body on meridians. The qi balances and increases in its flow through the meridians while you do qigong. The value of this is that the flows of qi in the body are subject to the same imbalance and stagnation that affect earth qi. It is this sluggish, or poorly balanced, qi that leads to a decline in health. At some point this tendency toward reduced health becomes a turning point and a critical contributor to disease and a downward-spiraling sense of well-being. Qi spreads throughout the body on twelve meridians, which carry the nourishing qi to every organ of the body. These flows are well documented and can be readily found on acupuncture charts. The pattern of the flows is one of nature's rules. Adjusting the flows to the cycles of tian qi and di qi is the work of qigong.

The Dan Tian

In addition to riverlike flows, qi also has a storage place in the body. Qi is stored in the dan tian. The dan tian is a center, like an energy pouch, three to four inches down from the navel and in the center of the pelvis. Qigong nourishes the flow to the dan tian, where qi is stored, and to the meridians, where qi is dispersed.

 Dan tian: The internal reservoir deep in the center of the pelvis where qi is stored, increased in amount and vibration, and then dispersed throughout the body.

Over time, two basic approaches to this process of increasing and balancing qi have evolved: the *wai dan* style and the *nei dan* style.

Wai Dan

The focus of qigong's wai dan style is the maintenance of the correct amount of qi in the body. The movements concentrate qi in the arms and legs through the practitioner's focused guidance. As qigong is performed, the qi gathers in and around the arms and legs. When it reaches the "spilling over" point, the fresh qi starts to flow throughout the body's qi meridians. This flow of qi clears obstructions, sluggishness, and imbalances. In so doing, it nourishes the organs, bones, circulation, skin, and the entire body. The qigong practices you will see demonstrated in *Qigong Basics* will draw from this side of qigong.

Nei Dan

The second aspect of qigong is nei dan—"internal elixir." This form of qigong is far more intricate, complex, and inherently challenging. It was originally part of the secret qigong practice that was passed along from master to disciple (not just student). This was the path of celibacy and enlightenment offered to, and embraced by, only a few. Rigorous and disciplined, nei dan focuses on the increase of the qi from within. From this internal center it is then dispersed throughout the entire meridian system to the arms and hands, legs and feet. Three types of qi circulation are used: water, fire, and wind. This form of qigong is best learned from an experienced teacher.

The type and quality of qi available to ren qi are influenced by a variety of natural factors. This elixir of life is affected by light—sunlight, moonlight, eclipse light, evening, dark, and so forth. The more light, the more active and intense the breath/qi. The softer light of the moon brings a corresponding change in the activity and intensity of the qi. Some forms of qigong are done in specific types of light.

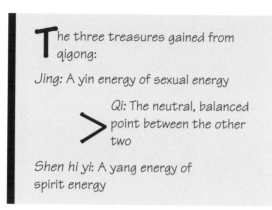

The three treasures gained from qigong:

Jing: A yin energy of sexual energy

Qi: The neutral, balanced point between the other two

Shen hi yi: A yang energy of spirit energy

When done in the correct series of movement and breath sequences, qigong creates an opportunity to reap valuable benefits. By allowing these concurrent elements to interact and achieve balance, qigong bestows three treasures upon the practitioner—the rewards of achieving balance between tian qi yang force and di qi yin, or feminine, force. When each type of qi is at its midpoint of balance, then the ultimate gift of each is accessible.

Di qi's balance brings depth and meaning, and intimacy, both sexual and empathic. Tian qi brings great spiritual intimacy, inner peace, and harmony. And qi, the balance or neutrality between them, brings equanimity.

The entire philosophy of qigong is breath as the elixir while the breath disperses throughout the body. Follow the ancient steps precisely in the qigong

Qigong may seem difficult at first, because you have to make yourself do it. Take heart. You will soon find your own rhythm.

of your choice, and you will be focusing your awareness to guide the qi to benefit yourself. As with all Eastern disciplines, the longer you do it, the higher the yield. Qi is a powerful force that may be invisible to the eyes of most, but is eminently recognizable to the body, which receives and absorbs it readily.

A qigong guide is useful. It allows you to avoid many areas of imprecise practice that would otherwise inevitably slow your own self-help process. Qigong has been beautifully crafted and polished over thousands of years to make it the effective system that is available to you today. To grasp all that it has to offer, it makes the most sense to stand on this venerable foundation with the support of an excellent teacher.

We can benefit from the wisdom of those who have achieved success in qigong before us:

Qi will bring warmth to the body and soul.

Qi will assist the emotions to be fluid and balanced.

Qi will show how to embrace life as a fluid process.

Qi will balance the polarities of energy—yin and yang.

Qi is found in air and oxygen as vital breath.

Qi permeates and surrounds all things natural.

Qi extends vitality.

Qi can be effectively supplemented with live food, meditation, and forays into nature.

Qi can be merged in sexual sharing.

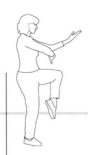

chapter 3

different forms
of qigong

ONE OF QIGONG'S great strengths is that it has grown into multiple forms born from a single root. The basics of qigong have been adapted, adjusted, honed, and developed to serve specifically desired outcomes. Qigong's ability to enhance all life makes it an asset in any endeavor.

The priorities of ancient China's culture cast the variations of qigong into three basic categories: medical, martial, and spiritual. Within these three categories the varieties of qigong were numerous. Each form was developed to support a specific arena of interest, with its own dedicated teachers, mentors, and students.

Very ancient, early people lived on the earth when the air was perfect. They lived here when light was not filtered through chemicals. They lived here when exercise was a part of life and when the inner-world connection between people was stronger and deeper than the outer-world connection. They were closer to the pulses of nature than we can imagine. From this pure environment of breath, light, and qi, qigong was probably born. People of that era didn't need to make time for movement. Movement happened naturally all the time. They weren't concerned about the body doing one thing and the mind doing another—most of the day the two were working in unison. They may have embodied qigong just in living their lives—who knows? What has been handed down to us today is a means of reinvigorating our bodies with the energetic health that is a prerequisite to any fulfilling life, a recipe for a more stable inner life that creates a richer and fuller outer life.

There were also great differences in the generosity with which qigong was shared. The forms that supported health and healing passed through the lay people of China and were endlessly imparted. It is from this branch that the popular qigong we know in the West was founded.

Martial arts qigong was shared throughout the training temples, but not beyond each temple's colony of highly disciplined monk/warriors. This attitude of concealment continued until the 1900s, when China's ancient structure began to relinquish its secrets to the rest of the world, and qigong was passed on. Martial arts qigong is generally known as chi kung, and is pronounced the same (qi/ chi = "key"; gong/kung = "gung").

Even today, qigong's ancient movements provide each practitioner the ability to upgrade:

Health and healing

Strength and self-preservation

Self-confidence and communication

Motivation and spiritual awakening

Add in an unbridled sense of personal well-being. This is internal security founded on the bedrock of an enduring truth—qi.

The qigong that was intricately crafted to support spiritual attainment was the most guarded, secretive form. Taught by master to disciple, some forms were shared throughout a monastery, but others were transmitted only to a chosen few. The good news is that all qigong movement arrives at the same place: improved health, greater skill in self-preservation, and well-being derived from spiritual attunement.

During its thousands of years of morphing, qigong has never lost its essential qualities. The root that nourishes all variations of qigong is the trained skill to direct the mind to qi. The disciplines of drawing qi into the body and increasing and cultivating qi join the beginner and the master—the difference is the skill with which the qi is controlled. To an observer, both seem to be moving in perfect, flowing unison, but the internal experience can be vastly different. One is simply learning the movements, while the other is in deep union with qi. It is this deep union that creates qi's enduring and inspirational impact on its practitioners. Qigong gently confronts all blockages to health and well-being and dissolves them.

Directing qi is the root essence of qigong. In the smoothly interactive components of mind-breath-movement, qigong practitioners achieve mastery over

"**S**pontaneous qigong"...
is an approach where we simply feel and follow the natural flow of our energy into whatever kind of movement feels right. In order to explore this more, take either the Earth and Heaven breathing or the Holding the Moon posture, and allow these exercises to be the themes upon which you, like a jazz musician, improvise. If this is enjoyable and comfortable for you, allow yourself to also explore vocalizing with the movement. Adding this element can be more emotionally evocative. Doing this kind of spontaneous qigong is inappropriate for those with unresolved emotional illness or trauma because it can be very powerful, so be sensible.

—Fernando Raynolds, Instructor
  Everything Tai Chi and
  Qigong Book

the essential nourishment of qi. The goal has always been consistently attainable through the daily use of qigong, no matter what variation was being practiced. This fact bears silent testimony to its nature as an inexhaustible indwelling fountain and to its multifaceted influence on life. Qigong still has the ability to deliver.

Three Forms of Qigong

The three forms introduced here are only examples of the wide variety of forms practiced.

The Eight Pieces of Brocade, or *ba duan jin*, 850 years old, is a form of qigong that is among the most widely practiced. It is considered an essential element in gaining understanding of our affiliation with qi. One story describing the beginnings of the Eight Pieces of Brocade, from the great collection of fact and lore that constitutes Chinese history, credits Marshal Yue Fe with it's creation.

Marshal Yue Fei, a renowned military commander born in the Song dynasty, developed the Eight Brocades (perhaps originally Twelve Brocades) to uplift the mental attitude and physical stamina of the common soldier. His role in bringing strength to the standards and values of China has left his memory revered.

Marshal Yue Fei lived through a time of war, corruption, and far too frequent famines. Through the steadfast application of his noble beliefs, he rose from peasant to high-ranking military officer. His successes and challenges were the stuff of timeless morality plays, novels, and biographies. After suffering a martyr's death, he became an eternal hero in the hearts of the Chinese people. It was his concern for his men's health and for safeguarding his nation's security that led him to create the Eight Brocades.

The version of the Eight Pieces of Brocade presented in this book is performed from a standing position and designed to be executed as softly and smoothly as silk brocade being moved gently by the breeze. This qigong is well suited to beginners and low-energy days. Eight Pieces of Brocade is taught by a variety of teachers, but certain basic similarities are common to all varieties. This form is inspired by Ken Cohen's book *The Way of Qigong*. (See chapter 14, "Eight Pieces of Brocade.")

A second qigong form, *t'ai chi ch'uan chi kung,* which comes from the t'ai chi ch'uan tradition, was developed centuries ago to support the martial arts. Master Tsung Hwa Jou presents it in his book *The Tao of T'ai Chi Ch'uan, Way to Rejuvenation*. Master Jou, at forty-seven, began t'ai chi ch'uan, practiced, and cured himself of an incurable illness. The strength of this personal healing set him on a life course of sharing and teaching t'ai chi ch'uan and qigong. It is through his teaching that this form of qigong is available today.

Qigong was an essential component to t'ai chi ch'uan because qigong provides a means to attain great internal strength. When the internal qi is smooth and balanced, the external force is graceful and powerful.

This style of qigong is done standing, with much arm movement. The legs move somewhat. The movements are coupled with the breath, and the two are coordinated with two sounds—*heng* on the inhaled breath, *haah* on the exhaled breath. The inhale is coupled with a contracting lower abdomen. The exhale is coupled with an expanding lower abdomen.

In Master Jou's own words: "A student will gain greater understanding of the three ingredients necessary for the mastery of this [T'ai Chi Ch'uan] art—balancing the chi and the blood building up inner energy and knowing the secret of T'ai Chi Ch'uan, which is T'ai Chi Chi Kung." (As has been mentioned, chi kung is another name for qigong, and both are pronounced the same.) (See chapter 15, "T'ai Chi Ch'uan Chi Kung.")

The third variation is Shaolin Si qigong. This form aligns the three major qi flows—tian qi, di qi, and ren qi. Their proper alignment produces a state of inner and outer harmony often associated with the aftermath of qigong practice. Harmony is a consequence of the effective direction of a component of qi—the five elements of wood, fire, earth, metal, and water. Follow the qigong movements and breath exactly—your qi will align as a matter of course.

Every form of qigong includes balancing the five elements. Shaolin Si qigong incorporates them; the Eight Brocades focuses on them. Qi and the five elements model is useful to understand as a part of learning any qigong form.

Qi—tian qi, di qi, and ren qi—is an intertwined web of life. Each component is a part of the whole, the dao. Wholeness could not exist without each component. Alter one component, and the entire web adjusts to reestablish balance.

Wu Hsing is a 2000-year-old theory of qi and the dao; it is a holistic approach to life based on the five elements. The five elements are understood to be nature's basic five components but are also seen as a dynamic process that is a vehicle for qi in its journey to nourish the body's organs.

Qi divides into the two basic components of life—feminine, yin, and masculine, yang. The two opposing but balanced forces refine further into the qi flows of the five elements. These divergent but interactive qi flows derive from the same dynamic process that characterizes the earth's elements. They are:

Wood • Fire • Earth • Metal • Water

It was determined that the five elements governed and were influenced by a great many aspects of the natural world.

In nature it is this dynamic process that destroys, regenerates, nourishes, and sustains the earth:

Wood creates fire (wood burns).

Fire creates earth (ash becomes soil).

Earth creates metal (found in earth).

Metal creates water (dew in the morning).

Water creates wood (nourishes plants).

And so it goes, round and round. When not interfered with, this circle of interaction provides all that nature needs to thrive, and nature is in balance.

Wood		Fire		Earth		Metal		Water	
yin	yang	yin	yang	yin	yang	yin	yang	yin	yang
liver	gall	heart	small	spleen	stomach	lungs	large	kidney	bladder
	bladder		Intestine				Intestine		

Table 3-1: The five elements and the qi nourishments of ten organs

	Wood	Fire	Earth	Metal	Water
Direction	East	South	Center	West	North
Season	Spring	Summer	Indian Summer	Fall	Winter
Organs	Liver	Heart	spleen	Lungs	Kidney
Colors	Blue	Red	Yellow	White	Black

Table 3-2: The elements and that which they govern

This five-elements process is mirrored in the human body. It works something like this: Tian qi empowers di qi as it enters the earth's field. Di qi divides into yin and yang. As yin and yang empower ren qi, they are refined into the five element flows. Each one of the flows, five yin flows and five yang flows, nourishes a specific organ in the body. The nourishing flow through the organs is a mirror of nature.

It is essential for good health to have the five-element qi flows moving through the body, nourishing their respective organs. Qigong is ideal for balancing and moving the five elements in a creative cycle so that each brings life and health to the next—the cycle of life.

This model of health emphasizes the interdependence of the organs rather than their individual function. Through the monitoring of the five elements, one can correct an imbalance in the qi flows.

Imagine a stream of water moving from a natural spring down a narrow channel. Growing all around the channel are a variety of plants dependent on this fresh, clear water for life. Occasionally a plant extends too far into the channel, impeding the flow of the water. This extension of root, moss, stems, and leaves slows or actually blocks the stream for the other plants downstream.

Now imagine further that you are gently drawing your finger through the spring water channel, from source to termination. As you gently move your finger through the water, you loosen the debris, and they float away and dissipate. You loosen roots, dislodge moss, and generally clean up the flow so it moves along for the benefit of all the dependent plant life of the entire system.

This is what we will be doing in the health qigong described in *Qigong*

---

*Q*igong practitioners traditionally have believed that:

Prevention is the best cure.

Medicine is mostly useful in curing disease.

Benefits of Balanced Qi:

Improved health

Radiant skin and eyes

Better metabolic rate

Deep and dreamless sleep

Increased physical strength

Improved mental focus

Appropriate emotional control

Increased intuition

Increased sexual energy

Basics. Qi, although usually invisible to the eye, is discernible through mental imagery. Qigong movement, coupled with breath and sound, is beautifully designed to clear the qi flows to the organs, the five element flows. Doing this qigong is like running a finger gently and slowly through the debris and unblocking your natural qi flow to restore clear, smooth qi movement. It is this clear movement that nourishes each organ and improves skin, strength, and general well-being.

Qigong has effective forms that require less memorizing of sequential flowing positions. More stationary, these forms focus on drawing in the breath, the carrier of the qi. As qi enters and is dispersed throughout the body, the energy meridians begin to balance through the yin and yang flow (you feel calmer). The reservoirs for the qi begin to fill (you feel more alive). The qi is now full enough in your body, and you can begin the qi cultivation process (you feel creative, with plenty of juice). As you cultivate the qi, the reservoirs of energy stabilize and fill the meridians (you have more energy to harness, and you can focus it). The meridians become plump and rich with qi. Yin and yang flows find their natural balance, given your temperament, and you feel at home and at peace with yourself. You may find your weight adjusts to your ideal body weight for maximum well-being. You may find yourself feeling that you have more time. You may find your simple pleasures in life becoming more intense. You may even find that you like, or even love, yourself and your life more than ever. I believe these are the natural birthrights of each one of us. We have created a culture that does not understand or appreciate the lasting benefits of a well-balanced life. There has been, until recently, very little support for achieving and maintaining health by means of the ancient wisdoms of breath, energy, intent, and self-discipline. Qigong has thrived all these thousands of years because, by its very nature, it returns us to these basic balances.

part 2
getting started

GETTING STARTED requires only one thing: just doing it. Reading this book is excellent preparation. Having a context within which to understand qigong, before actually beginning your lessons, brings greater depth and meaning to your practice. There comes a point when the shift from mental exploration to physical action is the only piece left to put in place.

Overcome any hesitancy. Don't over think it. Don't succumb to the belief that understanding it mentally is the same as taking part in the qigong experience. You are well prepared. Getting started is the next step in your sequence of learning. Let this chapter give you good support as you launch into your initial qigong practice.

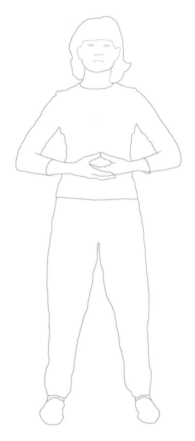

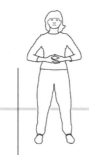

chapter 4

choosing the right form for you

CHOICE MAY SEEM like a quandary at this point. So many forms, too many choices. Take heart. All qigong styles lead back to a single beginning. All the basic theory, all the practice of this style or that, all the simple forms and the fabulously complex forms lead to the same place—the natural system upon which all life depends.

Any form of qigong will reveal the value of qigong practice. And this understanding enhances your commitment to the form, a path on which you join many, many others.

The Foundation of Qigong

The basic, unchanging foundation of every variation consists of: qi, meridians, dan tian, groundedness, quiet mind, repetition, deepening, integration, and providing time for the body to heal. No matter what form of qigong you choose, all of these elements will be present.

Qi

Understanding qi means coming into the realization that we human beings are an intrinsic part of the fabric of nature. We share qi with all of the earth's nature. Being open to developing this awareness will help you frame your new perceptions as they occur—for instance, when your senses become pleasurably heightened.

Meridians

Meridians are a network of channels that crisscross the body, moving from up to down, and from down to up. The contents of the channels, qi, is being transported throughout the body, providing needed nourishment to organs and balancing the yin and yang aspects of qi. Qigong movements and breath will show you how to open, regulate, and balance the meridians for your optimum health.

Dan Tian

There are actually three dan tians, but the basic one is deep in the pelvis. This is the energy center of the body, from which all qigong breath and movement emanate. The preference you may have for a very flat abdomen may change into a greater affinity for deep and complete breathing into the dan tian.

Groundedness

The "bubbling wells"—energy centers in the soles of the feet—make us aware of the ground as our foundation. This important energy center is down from the second toe to the bottom of the ball of the foot. There is an indentation that your finger can slide right into; this point roots the body energetically to the earth. All of qigong emphasizes the ground, the foundation for any form. Developing groundedness will give you a sense of self-acceptance and inner security.

Quiet Mind

The hallmark of qigong practice is the increasingly tranquil mind. A tranquil mind is not a passive mind. A tranquil mind, free of mental anxiety, is the master of correct timing, and correct timing will allow you to perceive the perfection in all of life.

Repetition

You will do the form or an aspect of the form over and over again. Because this is tedious at first, it will make you confront the depth of your commitment. However, the more you repeat, the more you will understand the need to repeat and the pleasure of repeating. The grounded structure developed by the repetitions becomes the basis for your understanding of all the subtleties of qigong.

As you practice, break up the monotony of repetition with questions:

How does my breathing feel?

Where in my body do I feel the breath?

Is the breath helping me move and balance?

How fast or slow is my normal breath?

Deepening

Deepening actually reveals that repetition is an illusion. To the outside observer, you are repeating, but as you "deepen into" the form, the sense of repetition will be replaced by a sense of ever-changing newness in the world of qi you are starting to explore ever more deeply.

Integration

Now your body has gotten the basics down, and they come to you automatically. The movement has deepened from the conscious to the unconscious mind. You are now able to feel the freedom in the movement and in your ever-deepening awareness as you move through conscious experience to the unconscious, as the unconscious opens and you are integrated into the whole fabric of nature. Your perceptions increase, and your sense of wholeness becomes a reality.

Providing Time for the Body to Heal

First you commit to doing qigong. Then you do it. Finally, after practice, you spend time letting your body rebalance and self-heal. This is the third essential component of a qigong triad for success. Qigong teaches the body self-healing. Do qigong, then stop everything and rest for ten or fifteen minutes. Then race back into life.

Every form of qigong you read about or actually do will contain these basic elements, consistently, throughout practice. When you explore new forms, these are the ever-present constants you can rely on.

Three Variations of Qigong

The form you choose often depends on the aspect of your life you have decided to enhance. As we've discussed, basic qigong forms fall into three general areas:

Martial qigong, to enhance strength, grace, and agility through strategic conflict

Spiritual qigong, to enhance spiritual attunement and advance on the path to enlightenment

Medical qigong, to enhance health and healing through the comprehension and guidance of qi

Of the three basic approaches to qigong, the forms growing the most quickly in popularity are variations on the medical form. This form works with qi alignment and direction for its own sake. The other qigong forms are designed to support another goal—martial arts for one and spiritual attainment for the other. Those orientations require more intricate crafting. Medical is a good place to start. Later, your growing affinity for qigong may lead you into other, more complex, forms and the goals with which they are aligned.

Categories of Qigong
Health maintenance
Healing
Longevity
Martial arts
Enlightenment

Whatever style you choose, the form is a blossom that draws from a common root. The forms shown in *Qigong Basics* are only three of many, many forms practiced. The form is less important than the mental strengthening, focusing, and directing of qi that belong to every style. This mental achievement is the common foundation.

As with anything, get the basics down and the rest is personal expression. The basic theory will bring clarity to the how, why, and what of essential qigong. And once you find your personal expression of the form, you'll find that the form becomes the teacher.

No matter the choice of form, it is essential to your health that you understand that qi exists in the body. Qigong provides a format in which to validate qi's existence. Your practice of qigong takes qi from theory to personal experience. You also need to have a clear and comprehensive visual image of the circulating paths of qi common to all human beings. Once you begin your practice, you will be embarking on a path that ensures the flowing circulation of your qi is sure, strong, and smooth.

 With this knowledge as a foundation . . . it will offer the beginner the key to open the gate into the spacious, four-thousand-year-old garden of Chinese Qigong.

—Dr. Yang Jwing-Ming, *Eight Simple Qigong Exercises for Health*

Your Choice

The three basic variations—martial, spiritual, and medical—offer you a choice. Which aspect of the triune do you want to emphasize?

The Basic Qis

1. Original qi (*xian tian qi*) is a prebirth qi that is attained from the parents at conception.

2. Post-birth qi (*houtian qi*) is the qi we draw in from air, food, and water

Qigong cultivates and directs both types of qi.

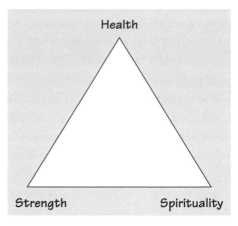

4-1: Three variations chart

The choice of the right form to start your qigong development is best approached through several avenues:

- Physical capabilities
- Personal orientation
- Class availability
- Quality of teacher
- Time commitment

Physical Capabilities

This tops the list, since qigong adapts so beautifully to any situation. Choose a form that complements your available range of motion. Some forms, such as Hwa's t'ai chi ch'uan chi kung (see chapter 15), adapt easily to sitting, or even lying down. The other forms in chapters 14 and 15 are involved with range of movement and shifting of balance. You will find as you faithfully repeat your chosen form that your range of movement increases. This brings a great sense of satisfaction and personal relief. Qigong repays your efforts with a feeling of being able to change your body, even after it seems to have developed a mind of its own.

Personal Orientation

This is a highly subjective area and really requires your own self-knowledge. Are you a strength-oriented person? This might mean that a qigong designed by the martial arts schools would be perfect. But maybe you want to learn more about relaxation. In this case, a form of qigong that emphasizes health and spiritual awareness might be the one for you (chapter 14). Or are you short on time? If you want something simple and effective, qigong designed for a quick alignment with your circumstances and rebalancing of your qi would be a nice fit (chapter 15).

 Whether you are agile as a cat or wheelchair-bound, the gifts, rewards, and challenges are the same. Qigong is a great leveler.

The versions of qigong identified here will help you determine the right course for you. Experiment first and then choose a form to settle into, so that you will already be familiar with your chosen form. Settle into it. Let the form become more and more familiar. Experiment with the forms suggested in *Qigong Basics*. Get familiar with them, pick your favorite, find the time, and practice daily. Then look to your community environment to expand your experience with a teacher. Even if this means learning an entirely new form, it won't matter. You will bring with you the nine constants of qigong: qi, meridians, dan tian, groundedness, deepening, integration, tranquil mind, repetition, and healing time. These nine aspects, inevitably a part of any practice, ensure that you will experience compatibility with any new form.

A student of qigong, an engineer, was taking qigong to improve his martial art of t'ai chi ch'uan. His interest was not in sensing qi. He had no interest, really, in qigong's ability to balance and enhance qi. He wanted to get stronger. However, as months, and then years, passed, he became more and more aware of the differences in energy fields around him. Precision was his nature, and eventually his ability to guide and direct qi astonished both himself and his teacher. This is a very interesting transition that often takes place. As people do qigong, even if they think the idea of qi is a fantasy, yet they will develop sensitivity to qi nevertheless.

Class Availability

If you have an idea of your area of primary interest, it is perfectly acceptable to contact a qigong center or teacher and have a talk. Ask about the form(s) they teach, the history of the form, and the orientation of the teacher—very important. Get a feel for what is being offered. Go for a trial class, test the waters, get a feel for the other students, the environment, and most importantly, the teacher. Then make your choice. It may be a match made in heaven right from the start, but if not—and you've given it six weeks—then move right on to another class. A calm and deliberate attitude will serve you best in your search for the class that meets your needs.

Quality of Teacher

Qigong must be learned from a teacher. A book can give you the lay of the land and get you started by giving you the most important information about qigong, but there can be no real progress without a teacher. The spoken word gives form and substance to the instructions. Everyone unconsciously favors or neglects some areas of the body. The keen eye of a skillful teacher can spot these uneven areas and make slight corrective adjustments to your performance of the form. These minor adjustments create major openings in the meridians and muscles. Without the teacher's observations, these openings may not occur. A teacher should have a history of studying with master teachers. It is these mentor relationships that continue the majestic tradition of qigong transmission. The lineage of mentor to student is essential for the practice of true qigong. Find a teacher who has learned from masters. Ask the orientation of the master and the orientation of the teacher. Does your teacher speak of the qigong master and the form with devotion and respect? Whatever form you choose, and then perhaps choose again, make sure that the exchange between yourself and the teacher demonstrates the quality of true qigong. If this isn't available to you, you are better off learning from a master on a video or DVD and periodically going to qigong seminar intensives.

Time Commitment

Love of qigong will produce a willingness, even a hunger, to commit the necessary time. But at first, the time commitment problem is the most frequently given reason for not continuing qigong practice. Embrace a form that fits easily into the niche of time you are allotting.

It makes no difference whether you do a simple form to completion or a portion of a more complex form. You don't need to do the whole form. Not at all. Pick a portion of the form, a sequence demonstrated by a picture or two. Pay close attention to the instructions. Pick a sequence you can easily remember, and then repeat it. Don't rush it. Settle into it. Make it fit your schedule. This is essential, otherwise you will feel pressed for time whenever you practice. What you want is a form or portion of a form whose sequence you settle into. The repetition provides the environment for the deepening to occur. This isn't about getting the whole thing

> Experiment first with the form.
>
> Find one you like.
>
> Stick with it.
>
> Keep it simple.
>
> Learn it.
>
> Repeat it.
>
> Deepen within it.

done—whew!—and hurrying on to the next thing. This is about a flower opening slowly. Let the form bring you into that pace. Pick your variation with this in mind. Then:

- Stick with that form for at least six weeks.
- Keep it simple so you can learn it.
- Repeat it again and again.
- Breathe and deepen.
- Find a teacher.

If you choose to go the evolutionary route, progressing from the simplest to the most complex forms of qigong, start with a health and well-being form. This will create internal strength and give you a great start on qi awareness. When you have reached a point of skill and competence, ask your teacher about studying t'ai chi ch'uan and the qigong associated with it. After many years of building skill on this second level, you will be ready for the Buddhist, dao, or Hindu qigong. Spiritual development is the most successful when the body is as healthy and strong as it is individually capable of being. Then the internal and external strength and discipline required to attain a state of enlightenment are fully integrated. Spiritual focus is most appropriate when you have reached that level.

We live in a "get it now" culture, but in China, life was tied to the seasons. Maturing was valued as a ripening of wisdom, and older people were revered for their warmth and wisdom. At that pace, it makes sense to leave one's spiritual qigong for the last step.

It makes sense in our country, too. All three aspects of the triune—health, strength, and spirituality—are active through each phase of life, but the first third of life is primarily focused on building up the body, the second third on

---

Three Treasures (San Bao)

Jing – Essence –
   Earthly essence

Qi – Internal energy –
   Body essence

Shen – Spirit –
   Mind essence

having the strength and stamina to live a full life, and the final third on developing the inner stillness of spiritual peace. No matter your age, it is still very much in harmony with qigong's rhythm to follow the same path. And if you have chosen your form with your needs in mind, you may find that your one form brings you the entire triune, through all the seasons of your life, to your complete satisfaction.

T'ai Chi and Qigong

You may be a bit confused about the difference between qigong and t'ai chi. To the casual observer they can appear quite similar. When you read about what each accomplishes, the basics seem at least similar, in some ways, and at times even indistinguishable. The ultimate contribution to health in both is based on the enhancement of qi. Essentially they are interwoven—qigong interwoven into t'ai chi.

Qigong is much older than t'ai chi and t'ai chi ch'uan. T'ai chi is a recent offshoot of t'ai chi ch'uan, which is a martial art that incorporated qigong into its martial art form. T'ai chi ch'uan, first and foremost, is about maintaining grace and form in a conflict situation. It also provides a route to health, well-being, and spiritual awareness.

T'ai chi ch'uan integrated qigong because it enhanced internal strength and universal connectedness. Qigong improved performance, enhanced courage, and empowered practitioners to perform greater feats. Qigong also continued to evolve among the Chinese people at large, as an integral movement of its own.

When t'ai chi ch'uan moved to the West, it softened. This flowing, light, softness was primarily created by Master Al Huang. As a child in China he watched t'ai chi ch'uan being performed not only as a martial form, but also as a movement for energetic balance. Today all over China, t'ai chi is performed in this way, individually and in small groups. A natural dancer, Master Huang brought his exquisite form of t'ai chi to the U.S. and taught it at Esalen Institute in Big Sur, California. There, he sowed the seeds for Western t'ai chi without the ch'uan martial aspects.

T'ai means supreme. *Chi* mean ultimate. *Ch'uan* means fist. T'ai chi drops the fist, but retains some martial moves. Pushes and kicks are common in t'ai chi forms.

Qigong has no martial component. The moves are crafted to engage qi, expand its healing potential, and align the practitioners with universal nature.

Freedom to Choose

What all this really boils down to is that you have absolute freedom to pick whatever form appeals to your senses. This choice will be dictated somewhat by the availability of qigong instruction in your area. Videos and books are readily available. It is not difficult to learn the basics of the forms, but eventually you will want an instructor. The personal guidance and the mentor relationship are essential to perfecting the form and achieving a lasting experience of qigong's positive influence.

What if you find yourself ready for a teacher, and the form you want to learn isn't being taught? That is a disappointment, but remember—your ability to draw from qigong will remain unaltered. Remember, an enormous variety of qigong forms is being offered now. Choosing one does not mean lifelong loyalty to the form and the mentor. Dip into the forms and try a few. When you find the form that seems right, then settle into it.

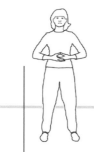

TEACHERS are definitely the most direct route to competence in qigong practice. The best guide is someone who has gone a little further down the road and is willing to share what he or she has learned along the way. This route to effectiveness has been particularly well mapped out in the teaching and learning of qigong—an ancient discipline that has been honed to its essence through the contributions of thousands. The teaching in this case is not so much a matter of verbal instructions from the teacher followed by the student's attempt at the motions—but rather a natural continuation of the long tradition of handing on qigong skills to the next generation of practitioners.

> In the China of old, qigong was taught to ill people, and this practice has continued up to the present day. The qigong mentor is a highly skilled practitioner who can demonstrate a specific qigong form to offset a body imbalance that is causing illness. No one is turned away. As long as qi moves within, there is a form that can be taught. If the patient can only wiggle a big toe, then that is where the form starts. Qigong is for anyone, whatever their ability to move.

How Qigong Is Taught

Qigong, learned more through example than through instruction, is most effective when practiced in an atmosphere where silence predominates. Unlike the Western approach to transferring information, which always includes a lot of verbal support, commands, analysis, or observations, the Eastern approach relies on a triune of communication: your qigong mentor, you, and qi.

Qigong, born of the people of China, moved through the generations, from

The value of the mentor has slipped in our competitive, youth-oriented culture. Old cultures have a place for the mentor-learner relationship. China leads in this. China lifted the role of the accomplished one, the sage, to a position of very great honor. Inherent in the culture was a responsibility the master carried to pass on his skill. This duty was deeply entrenched in the culture—the obligation to pass along what one had learned in a lifetime of commitment.

Making money is an essential component of our culture. That said, qigong mentors should have their love of qigong in balance with their need to make money at it. If money is your mentor's main reason for teaching, move on.

grandparent to parent to child. The transmission happened primarily through visual observation, rather than verbal guidance. This atmosphere of silence thrives in the mentor tradition. Historically, the mentor tradition of transmission dominated all three aspects of qigong. Concealed transmission, master to disciple, was the order of the day for the temples of faith and martial arts. Medical, or health and healing, qigong radiated throughout China in a tradition of free sharing. In the martial and spiritual forms of qigong, the one-to-one teacher and student or disciple tradition was the method of transmission.

In the spiritual and martial forms of qigong, you will generally find instruction taking place in a relaxed class format. Qigong is easily shared in this situation, students watching the teacher, fitting the breath into the movement as well as they can. The teacher then comes over with a gentle adjustment or quiet word. Teacher, student, and qi then become equals in the experience. The student "feels" qigong more personally. Eventually the teacher is no longer needed, for the student and the qi are together, and qigong is the result. When this balance has been found, the qigong practitioner is moving in obvious, graceful unison with qi. A good teacher is in the picture only to facilitate this, never to compete with qi for attention. With a few guidelines, you can choose your teacher/guide wisely. You can find someone whose process and goal is to free you for your own experience.

Qualities of a Good Teacher

A guide to finding a great mentor:

1. The practice of qigong is supposed to be a lifelong commitment.

2. Choose your mentor well. You want a mentor whose final goal is for you to be completely self-empowered, free to perform qigong as an act of union between you and qi.

In old China, the master was the pinnacle of years of focused achievement, living in a very structured, hierarchical subculture—a martial arts temple or a Buddhist monastery. The subculture provided safeguards against unwise teaching, so unquestioning obedience to the master was expected. These safeguards are not in place in our culture. If a qigong teacher asks you to do, accomplish, or take on a discipline that feels clearly wrong, question the teacher's authority. If your teacher is having ego and control issues, you do not serve the teacher's personal growth by following blindly.

1. Look for a mentor who has no personal need for followers. The class teaching style will be set up to return the student to his or her own inner guide. The mentor will guide and direct, but not dominate the student's inner voice. The mentor will not claim to be the final authority, but instead will embody humility as a result of the alliance with qi.

2. A mentor's sense of personal identity should not be limited to "teacher." Find a person who is able to sustain a comfortable balance between the teaching/mentoring "I know" identity and the sharing "we find out together" personality. This is consistent with the qigong value of balance.

3. A mentor's relationship to the learners should be supportive and respectful.

4. Your qigong teacher is a spiritual teacher of sorts. Spiritual teachers demonstrate their own evolution by embracing both their humanity and spirituality, together. A satisfying personal life in combination with a committed spiritual practice is the goal.

5. The mentor's commitment to sharing qigong should be untainted by an undercurrent of need for a closer personal association. Qigong is a full, complete learning process. It takes full concentration, and a mentor who has an underlying agenda can interfere with the learner's experience.

6. The mentor teaches the traditional movement and breath sequence and shares tried and true wisdom, not personal opinions.

7. You should feel empowered when you leave the mentor. Shame, comparison, or humiliation should never be a part of your learning experience.

8. Your mentor should have an ongoing relationship with a qigong master who is guiding her or him. This relationship ensures your mentor's ongoing development.

9. In watching your mentor execute the sequence, you should see a demonstration of exquisite movement. Simply watching should allow you to intuit the internal state of connectedness derived from the close association with qi.

10. Choose a mentor who takes time to explain the basics of qi and qigong. Explanations of the theory of qi, its movement, and the three treasures derived from qigong—jing, qi, and shen—create a helpful context for your inner experience as a learner.

11. Choose a mentor who can demonstrate and direct the regulation and guiding of the mind.

12. Choose a mentor who has found his or her own wellspring of qi. This is a silent knowing that is either present or absent. It is not control or detachment. It is the warmth of true connection.

13. Choose a mentor well versed in breath regulation and guidance.

14. Choose a mentor who understands, unequivocally, that unless these cornerstones of qigong are securely in place and well developed, there will be no deep appreciation of qi and its distribution.

15. Choose a mentor who teaches the form you are the most interested in.

Why are these standards so high? You are venturing into a field of connecting with qi more directly. In this sphere, the character of your mentor will affect you deeply. Sharing in the qi as the transmission occurs is an intimate experience.

> Qigong is a lifelong commitment. Your qigong mentor is a lifelong student, always learning, growing, and deepening in the form.

> If you successfully choose a good mentor and the form is a good fit, you will find qi awareness. This is a wonderful step in self-knowledge, good health, emotional well-being, and spiritual recognition.

Great teachers have filled human history with inexhaustible spiritual nourishment. Circumstances alter, cultures change, weather provides challenges, the cycle of gain and loss goes on and on, but the words of the masters prevail. They draw their wisdom from the qi.

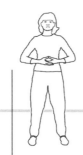

finding
the right class

A GOOD FORMAT for learning is *the* essential component for progress. A class is the most common Western format and is a fine, accepted way to learn. The learning proceeds more comfortably if certain elements are in place. These are the most basic elements:

A large class may interfere with the impact of learning from your teacher. One-to-one teaching can improve this situation.

Your format for learning is a choice for you alone. Reading a book to learn the form and then doing solitary practice is one format. Buying a video to follow along with is another. A one-to-one student-mentor alliance is another useful learning format. Joining a group in the park doing qigong for fun and just following along is yet another.

1. The class offers the form you are interested in. (A well-trained instructor goes without saying.)
2. The class is situated in a pleasant environment.
3. The class size is easily manageable.
4. The qigong mentor is easily visible and very engaged in teaching as well as doing qigong.
5. There is ample space to move around.
6. The lighting is soft and preferably not overhead.
7. There is good air movement, preferably fresh air.
8. Your mentor takes time to warmly welcome each student to class. This sets the tone of the class and ensures the open attitude essential for qi awareness.

Choosing the Right Class Format for You

In addition to the basics, there are other components of a class that can enrich your learning experience. The more of these elements a qigong class offers, the richer the environment for learning the form you have chosen.

A class fee is usual in Western practice. It is a case of the students providing for the teacher, so the teacher can provide for the students.

A Relaxed Yet Well-Structured Class

Generally, class time extends from about forty-five minutes to one and a half hours. The class should provide ample time to relax, focus, learn, and integrate the new material with what you have learned before. Generally, a sequence of learning is something like this:

Enter.

A moment is taken to honor the lineage of qigong masters.

Stretch, loosen, and relax to prepare for qigong.

Perform warmup movement and breath work.

Perform the qigong movement, as one flowing sequence up to the last sequences taught.

The next step in the sequence is demonstrated by the mentor, first verbally and then as a movement.

Then the entire sequence is repeated, with the new sequences added in.

Students focus on learning the new sequence.

The entire sequence is repeated with the new sequences added in.

The form is again repeated, and this time the focus is on the element of breathing.

Meditation time is given to integrate the effects of the class into your repertoire.

A moment is taken to honor the lineage of masters.

Class is dismissed.

The Class Is Situated in a Pleasant Environment

Nature is best. That said, building-enclosed classes are more common. Qigong thrives in an atmosphere of happy, balanced qi. Perhaps more than other forms of movement, qigong is vulnerable to the qi environment in which the qigong movement takes place.

Qigong form is like a window. It provides a frame in which to better see beyond the window's structure. Qi is the view that flows to you through the window.

Qigong draws qi in and distributes it throughout the body. Qi is either harmonized or disrupted by the environment through which it flows. Qigong blurs the boundary between the outer qi fields and the inner qi field of the body. In the blurring of this boundary, many wonderful events occur.

The body fills with more qi.

The practitioner feels a sense of connection to the universe.

The qi flows of yin and yang balance.

The organs of the body receive nourishment.

Health blossoms.

Qi creates a condition in which the inner qi flows balance with the outer qi flows.

This last one is the reason the class environment should be appropriate. Let's face it—there are some environments with which we would not want to harmonize. There is an expectation, and rightly so, that a qigong class will provide an environment in which harmonizing is beneficial, centering, healing, and complete. To achieve this, the environment should employ the art of natural or designed feng shui. Generally, nature is qi in balance, and rooms are not.

There are many areas where qi, which should flow like a river, meets obstacles, such as stairs, sharp corners, or dead ends, causing it to rush too fast, pile up, and/or stagnate. Qigong, designed to draw in and balance qi, will draw in these out-of-balance flows. The qigong movements will succeed in balancing them within, but not without effort. It is better to be in harmony to begin with. Qigong in a harmonious environment ensures maximum communion with the gentle sweetness offered by earthly and heavenly qi.

As qigong is opening you to the qi field around you, nature is your best bet. Performing qigong on the grass (especially with dew underfoot), among bushes, flowers, and trees, is always beneficial.

An inside class requires some careful placement of items to imitate what nature offers naturally. The Chinese practice feng shui, the art of correctly analyzing the relationship of the elements within a location, especially the relationship between wind and water and their reaction to the terrain in which they flow. Once the flowing patterns are understood, placements can be made that will alter the flows.

Feng shui teaches the art of placement to enhance the smooth flows of qi. Specific elements—water, minerals, fire, mirrors, flowers, plants, mounds of earth, fresh air, and more—are combined uniquely and wisely to create a harmonious flow of qi. Qigong provides the balance within, and feng shui balances the environment without.

If the class is inside, the flows of qi will respond to the dimensions and building design of the room. It is a gift to everyone if the instructor has used wise placement of specific elements to enhance the room's balance. There are many books on feng shui available to guide and direct the arrangement. It need not be complex. Elements can include:

- A small water fountain
- A plant
- A fan to gently stir the air/qi
- Fabric to soften the corners
- A light to soften and focus the qi
- Flowers to enhance and soften the atmosphere

Each element, carefully placed, has a simultaneously subtle and powerful effect. The space will define the feng shui needed. A wise instructor takes time to align a classroom prior to each class.

A Supportive Emotional Environment

Although invisible to most, qi is still felt by most. Qi communicates its presence in nonverbal ways. A sense of warmth, a feeling of increased body comfort, a decrease in pain, or an adjustment in a tight area may be your internal intelligence discerning qi—its presence and its effects, all of which lead toward improved health

Why is a silent, qi-harmonious environment so emphasized?

We have designed a culture of amazing opportunities, but one with very little emphasis on the value of qi. Qigong classes provide an oasis in a rushed life. To the degree that the class environment is one in which qi is nourished, the constant pressures of our life will find relief.

and well-being. The qigong form is taught to sensitize you to your qi awareness. Intuition shows you how to proceed with your accumulating knowledge.
The wisdom of your mentor is essential for efficient learning of the form, but
your own intuition is your personal language for communicating with qi. Any
good class will support the developing intimate relationship between you and
qi. This type of class orientation will support your personal pace of learning.
This type of class will also continually remind you that less effort is the way to
true qigong.

Timing

Timing is everything. Commitment is timing's sibling. Decide on your class
time according to these considerations:

1. It has to be a reasonable, manageable fit with your schedule.
2. The will to commit is essential.
3. There will be class time and practice time.

At first it will be an effort, but as qigong gets under your skin, a change will
occur. Instead of forcing yourself to take the time for qigong and using will to
create commitment, you will discover a correlation between desire to do
qigong and having the time for it. The time will be there, and from that point
on, the quest for the time recedes. Qigong becomes a part of essential life. You
will have your own schedule.

Qigong will teach you about right timing in life in general. You will develop
an instinct for when to move forward or back and when to be neutral. Timing
is everything. Finding your place in timing is an essential requisite for a life
well lived.

Other Factors

Breath and Qi

Breath is the conveyor of qi. Qigong is
breath work perfectly aligned with specific
movement to enhance a specific outcome.

To this end, movement and breath are
taught as one unified element. The environment provides a good source of oxygen,
fresh and flowing. If the room is enclosed,
a fan should be well placed to ensure that

M ost people nor-
mally breathe
with great restriction.
There is no point in
emphasizing breath
work forms until abso-
lutely correct breath-
ing has become a way
of life. True normal
breathing alone brings
enriched health.

There are two basic types of qi-balancing forms:

Yin (passive) on the inside
Yang (active) on the outside

> Qigong movement with inner quiet and peace

Yang (active) on the inside
Yin (passive) on the outside

> No physical movement, active inner awareness

Doing both each day generates greater yin/yang balance.

the qi is not stagnating. Fresh water is essential, from either a source there or one you have brought with you.

Much time is spent initially on the experience of plain old normal breathing before progressing on to other forms of breath.

Focusing the Mind

Movement, breath, and mind are taught as an entwined triune on which qigong depends. Much useful time is spent focusing on the mind's guidance of the coordination of breath and movement. This includes focusing on a body part, drawing the qi to that part, and dispersing the qi throughout, with intent to nourish and heal. Qigong abounds in forms to facilitate this ability to guide the qi.

Meditation Session

Meditation is far more than sitting cross-legged with the eyes rolled up and in. Qigong opens the door to the gifts of meditation. Peace of mind, a sense of connection with the universe, increasing clarity, and personal awareness are the consistent results of meditating. Meditation is the perfect completion to any class.

Qi Distribution and Dispersal

This portion of the class is, by necessity, verbal. The mentor will introduce the Chinese theory of the five elements.

Diagrams of the qi meridians and their predictable flows through the body are thoroughly explored.

There are many formats for meditation:

☞ Sitting

☞ Walking

☞ Movements like qigong and t'ai chi

☞ Focusing completely on whatever is being done

☞ Breath release

☞ Chanting

There is a format to suit every person.

Time is taken for self-massage. Reflex areas are identified, brushing the meridians is exemplified, and massaging acupressure points is explored.

The meridians' link to the reason for qigong movements is explained.

Your Qigong Mentor Has a Newsletter

This newsletter has a vast amount of enriching information. Referrals to books, philosophical reflections, meditation techniques, nutrition, quotes, teaching tidbits, and information on the extended qigong community can be found here. The vast world of qigong that would otherwise be shared verbally, and somewhat disruptively, is instead imparted through the written word. These newsletters can then be passed along to others for their benefit.

No Class in Your Area?

1. Buy a video.

2. Invite a friend to join in.

3. Take a trip to study with a teacher.

4. Have a teacher come and do a weekend seminar.

5. Go to a qigong retreat.

6. Subscribe to a qigong magazine.

7. Remember, qi is awaiting you. You only need to embrace its reality and define your relationship with qi.

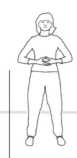

chapter 7
your first session

YOU HAVE CHOSEN your class and your teacher with care, and now you are ready for your first session. There are some practical steps you can take prior to the class that will promote its success.

Adopt a Learner's Attitude

A learner's attitude is the environment you bring to qigong. Qigong offers a tremendous advantage: you can benefit from thousands of years devoted to

---

The most important environment is inside you. So no matter whether you have a plethora of classes to choose from or only one you're stuck with, you have complete authority over your inner environment, which is where the successful learner's attitude begins and ends.

---

discovering the best methods for developing and directing qi. Thus the outcome of learning qigong is predictable—health improves, greater well-being is a constant, and a sense of wholeness permeates living. This is the consistent exit point, when you step out of the form.

The entrance point, however, is the human condition—stressed, depressed, sad, ebullient, angry, accepting, raging, shocked, lonely, supported, fulfilled, empty—the list is as endless as life itself. Qigong is open to one and all. The entrance point of the form embraces young and old, well and ill, serene and worried. There is no human dilemma or condition that can daunt qigong. Step into the form as you are, bring it all to the form, and the entrance point of improvement remains eternally open. Qi works with you as you engage the

Learner's Attitude

Every aspect of a form assumed within the qigong sequence has its own specific purpose and contribution to the whole. A learner commits to experiencing and understanding the root meaning of each aspect of the form.

Qigong Attitude

Will power

Gentle self-patience

Ability to be there no matter the weather

form and your sense of unity is restored. Your stage of learning has no effect on the outcome. You always feel better. The degree of improvement is what changes, growing greater and deeper as you progress in the form. The right environment to bring to qigong is you. A learner's attitude is one of gratitude to the many who have brought this dance of life to you. Humble, open, willing, and fully yourself—the qigong learner's attitude.

There are many ways you can prepare yourself, mentally, emotionally, physically, and spiritually, to enter the form. Here are a few. You will divine many more.

1. When stress pops up, say, "I'm sure looking forward to qigong later!"
2. After qigong I will do _____ (something you are looking forward to).
3. Focus on one area—your hand, for instance. Direct qi into your hand with your mind. and see if you can get your hand to warm up.
4. When you feel overly emotional, take a moment to realize that qigong will relieve the overload.
5. Take half an hour before class to focus on relaxing into normal breathing, while you do whatever you are doing.
6. Walk as if you are floating.
7. Move your arms as if qi is moving them from the inside.
8. Walk with awareness that you are not walking through emptiness, but through a vibrant qi field.
9. Initiate movement from the dan tian.
10. Bend your knees slightly. Relax your dan tian, exhale, release down. Inhale, draw earth qi, di qi, up from the Earth and through your legs, circulating it at the dan tian. Let your legs and pelvis get heavy, like a mountain. Now move your torso and arms lightly, as if being moved by a gentle wind.
11. Sit quietly and focus on an element of nature. Inhale air and qi, and then

Principles to Cultivate and Learn through Qigong:

1. Be natural, quiet, and relaxed.
    Find a place that is quiet, and calm yourself.

2. Combine the will and the qi.
    Focus your will and awareness on your breath.

3. Establish solidity in the lower body and legs.
    Fill both legs with earth energy.

4. Move slowly, and cultivate stability.
    Be steady and assured in your movements.

5. Practice diligently and regularly.
    Find a time that works in your busy life.

6. Observe moderation in the extent of movement.
    Don't force yourself into movement you are not ready for.

— Thanks to *The Tao of T'ai Chi Ch'uan*, by Jou Tusung Hwa

exhale, sending the qi in a flowing current back to nature. Sense the touching and merging. Arrive at a feeling of neutrality. The breath breathes you, and you dissolve into the breath.

A few additional ideas:

1. High-quality aroma essences abound, essences designed to effectively, even magically, influence mood, emotional state, and attitude. You know your stress vulnerabilities. Aromas that can have a favorable impact on your learner's attitude are available.

2. It can be useful to take time for self-care prior to or immediately after qigong. Massage, reflexology, acupuncture, facials, and more, all enhance the qigong state of being.

3. Flowers are an eternal source of mood enhancement. Just looking at flowers as you sprint past them can promote the correct learner's attitude.

4. Sit quietly, sense the qigong lineage—the masters and the ordinary people you are joining in shaping the evolution of qigong.

To promote inner quiet you might consider cutting back on caffeine. One possible reason for misuse of caffeine is the craving for the bitter flavor. Chinese medicine believes in getting a full variety of flavors—sour, sweet, salty, pungent, and bitter. We have a dearth of bitter flavors in the Western diet, but greens, asparagus, celery, hops, vinegar, and mineral supplements can help fill the need. If you satisfy your bitter craving elsewhere, your need for coffee and tea may decrease.

Clothes

You will feel the most comfortable wearing lightweight, fairly loose-fitting clothes that allow freedom of movement. Ideally, qigong is done in bare feet, but in our culture shoes are generally worn. T'ai chi cloth shoes provide a non-slip sole and light fabric body to enclose the foot. These can be slipped into any lightweight shoe, which makes them convenient for those who do better with arch supports. Lightweight running shoes work, as do slipper-type shoes, as long as they are not prone to sliding.

The color of the clothing you wear will have an effect on the qi. Whatever color you wear will add its essential quality to the overall effect qigong will have on you. Some colors are useful:

Red – Vitality

Orange – Physical strength

Green – Manifesting skill

Blue – Nurturing

Violet - Relaxation

White – Clarity and emanating

Black – Absorbing and integrating

Pink – Love and boundaries

Turquoise – Adaptation

Purple – Authority

Indigo – New ideas

Tan – Internal control

Brown – Grounding

You may very well find that the teachers and students in your chosen class are all wearing similar clothing, often black. Sometimes the teacher is affiliated with a specific qigong group or teacher and wears an outfit expressing this. These variations on the theme are not relevant to you as you begin—to not know is a beginning, and beginnings are thrilling. You have a whole world ahead of you. Don't get caught up in feeling out of place because of your concern over your clothes. Come comfortable, and know nothing—a beginning. Your primary concern in dressing for qigong is ease of movement, ease of breathing, and good support from non-slip shoes. If you are a bit unsteady, check with a professional to learn what footwear would be the most stable for you. Natural, simple, free-flowing, and secure that's it.

The Start of Class

Leave yourself plenty of time to get to the class. Even arrive a little early. This facilitates the calm inner mind that will be receptive to the class and its contents. But if life has other plans and you arrive ruffled and late, then that is the way it is. Qi still surrounds you. Breath and qi still move within you. Draw back your mind. Concentrate on your breath. Take a few good dan tian breaths. Leave the previous moments behind. Release.

Often qigong instructors greet new students personally. Don't be surprised if your teacher seems happy to have you in the class and welcomes you with a smile, introducing you to the group. Whether shy or outgoing, receive the greeting with grace and simplicity.

Note Your Progress

Form the habit of noticing your progress through the realization that stressed areas are softer and warmer. Aches can be dissolved. You are more able to reverse the body's tendency to store stress. Take a brief moment at closure to appreciate the form and the many masters who have gifted you with their skillfully crafted art.

Situate Yourself

Locate a spot in the class where you can easily see the instructor. Or, the instructor may guide you to a spot. Here are some things to watch for.

- Can you see clearly?
- Is the light conducive to seeing easily (i.e., it is not behind the teacher)?
- Can you move without concern for bumping into someone or something?
- Is the air free-flowing and not stuffy?
- Can you hear easily, or should you be closer?
- Where will you sit if you get tired?
- Where is the restroom?
- Have you taken off your wristwatch and jewelry?

Ground Yourself

Do a few preparatory stretches:

- Drop those roots from the bubbling well, deep and wide.
- Elevate your head, lifting the spine up, sword from a sheath.
- The pelvis and legs are grounded like a mountain.
- Your torso, arms, shoulders, neck, and head are as light as a breeze.
- Settle your mind onto your breath.
- Breathe from the dan tian, expanding the abdomen on the inhale, relaxing back to flatten it on the exhale.
- Relax, let your entire body sink downward, joints open and relaxed.
- As the inhale rolls through you, envision qi rising fountain-like from the dan tian, flowing up your torso, through the shoulders, down the arms, and out the fingers. Let your arms float up, buoyed by the qi. Then let your arms float down to your sides. Be in your dan tian breath.
- Relax within your form.

  Now you are ready.

Opening Ritual

Qigong classes sometimes start with a moment of appreciation for your teachers, master teacher, and for all who have gone before, leaving a trace of themselves in the sequences. This is very appropriate for several reasons. It can be a moment of thanks to previous masters. It can also be a brief moment to collect oneself and become fully present. Music may be turned on; a water fountain may be started; candles may be lit. There are many options. In this moment you are aligning yourself with qi, with your intent to do qigong, and opening into the form. This ritual of coming to the present and into the class experience is very important. It creates the space for qigong to flourish. It puts your experience into perspective—you are standing on the wisdom of all who have gone before.

It also puts the teacher into perspective. There is a tendency in qigong for some teachers to act as if they are the beginning and the end. Taking a moment to appreciate the previous generations puts this teacher in the proper context. No matter how great, the teacher is just one player in a very large team. Humility is a good quality for your teacher to express.

Finally, this time of appreciation is useful for your learning. Since we live in and are formed by a competitive culture, the desire to impress the teacher, to do it "right" and be the best beginner in the class is all too natural. This can interfere with your receptivity to the transmission of the form. See your teacher leading the class, and then imagine many other friendly teachers of the past standing behind your teacher, all of them there before your inner eye. Appreciate their contributions and your teacher's, and allow yourself to fill with appreciation. Appreciation equalizes, and you will be back in the flow of presence, competition and insecurity now receding into the past.

Your long-term goal is to do qigong well on your own. This should be your teacher's goal, too.

This sense of appreciation may create an awareness of what is meant by "stepping into the form." The ancient form is like a river that flows through long-established channels of movement. You become sensitized to the feeling of entering something previously established, something that has always been there. Joining into the breath, movement, and qi brings a sense of steadfast support and an experience that can be returned to again and again. Beginner and great master are equal in the form. The movement, when done in a group, exposes the flowing oneness gained by stepping into the form. Joining into the movement of omnipresence or qi carries inherent gifts of balance and joy. This probably won't be your dominant experience in the first or even the twentieth class, but it will come, and when you are there, when you and qi become one through qigong, you will understand and be filled with gratitude.

During Class

By this time, you will have practiced the sequences shown here in *Qigong Basics*. You will be familiar with the concept of moving out, so returning to center will not be entirely new to you. Your teacher will show you some beginning movements. Knowing the basics of grounding through bubbling well points will serve you well.

Enjoy watching others. Resist concerns that you won't ever be able to do that. Your time will come. As these concerns arise, concentrate on your breath. Take a dan tian breath or five, and get your mind under control by becoming present in your breath.

If you begin to feel faint, sit down immediately or lean against a wall. The faintness most likely occurs because your breath depth and movement are not in balance yet. If the problem persists, check with your doctor.

Often qigong increases the need to use the restroom. Know ahead of time where it is, and quietly exit when you need to. There are qigong teachers who do not allow bathroom breaks. If yours is one of these, my advice is to move on—no one wants to have a tyrant for a teacher.

Usually the class starts with an opening into the form and warmups. The warmups are straightforward, and I don't imagine they will give you a problem. But if they are strenuous, or you are recovering from an injury, don't push yourself. You will then move into your qigong sequence. The actual practice will depend upon what type of class you are in. There are two types. The first is a series of classes, usually six to ten sessions, set up for beginners. Everyone starts at the same place. This can be very useful. It makes learning the new steps peer-supported and fun. A beginning class will progress from the warmup to a basic presentation of the qigong stance, some breath work, and some movements with qi in mind. After the series of sessions is over, an intermediate class is next.

Do not do any qigong movements if you have health issues or injuries. High blood pressure or lower-back pain are some examples. Check first with your physician to get an O.K.

Points to keep in mind:

☞ Relax and settle downward.   ☞ Never lock the joints.

☞ Float through the movements.   ☞ Practice daily.

The second type of class is ongoing, and beginners are mixed in with other students of varying degrees of accomplishment. This class can be absolutely wonderful or it can be an intimidating nightmare. It will depend entirely on the teacher. You will know after your first session if this mixed class is for you. If it is confusing or intimidating, talk to your teacher. There may be other class alternatives. If not, don't be disheartened. You can:

• Look for another class
• Buy a good video
• Keep with it for a while to see if it gets better

A class like this can be a good environment for going at your own pace and personalizing qigong for yourself. If the teacher doesn't have time or interest for your concerns, exhale and move on.

An ongoing class will:

- Demonstrate the form up to the last thing learned
- Put in a new step
- Practice the new step

The teacher will determine where and how the beginner will join in the routine.

Generally, a qigong class lasts from about forty-five minutes to an hour and a half. When the class is over, there is often a completing ceremony. This may take the form of another salutation to the qigong lineage. It may be a moment of silence. It may be an emphasis on the completion of the form. This is a very important part of qigong. It closes down what was opened at the beginning of class. It punctuates the end of the class time. Your teacher will most likely want to find out how your initial experience was and whether you have any questions. If homework for practice hasn't been specifically outlined, this is a good time to ask for something to practice over the following week. You could also mention reading this book and ask for a recommendation for another book to read and a video to follow at home. Many teachers have their own companion video already produced. This helps a lot.

After Class

Now the class session is over. There will be silence, at first, as people adjust to the effect of the movement on them—a slightly altered state. Just take one action at a time in getting ready to leave, and you will be grounded when you exit. It is nice, if you live in a safe area, to take a qigong walk. The natural gait of walking is a way to integrate and balance the session's effects on and in your body. Appetite varies. It is better to go into class a bit hungry, but not with low blood sugar. After class, once the qi has balanced, you will most likely be hungry. Eat fresh foods filled with qi, and drink good, clear water. Often qigong will improve the quality of your sleep. You might sleep deeply and wake very refreshed. Plan to do a few qi breaths upon awakening.

For the second session, prepare as before, and you may want to add in an orienting inspiration. Bring it to the class and use it as the lens through which you engage the qigong. Any inspirational phrase you enjoy would be suitable. For example:

- Life is Love.
- Touch life gently.
- That was. This is.
- Fill with wonder.
- Seek what the masters sought.
- Qigong is self-love.

You can also retain an image of nature—movement like a breeze through leaves, grounded as a mountain, earth and heaven breathing together. Inspiration is everywhere, and the right one can add a beautiful dimension to qigong. Enjoy.

The practice of qigong can promote wonderful health, but the gifts of qigong won't be effective unless you take care of yourself.

Good food

Adequate rest

Exercise as a part of life

Add qigong to these three cornerstones of your health foundation, and you are committing to the benefits of qi.

Support for Qigong Success

Walking to balance body and energies

Acupuncture on a regular basis

Intent to manage emotions

Warming-up breath awareness

Excellent diet

Morning wellness workout

A few minutes for contemplation and gratitude

part 3

learning the basics

A MASTER OF ANY DISCIPLINE will say the same thing about his or her ability: the strength comes from knowing and returning time and again to the basics. Basics provide the needed foundation on which to build a successful relationship to qigong. And qigong's ancient traditional skills provide something else as well: powerful positions and breath maneuvering that have the ability to mysteriously align the practitioner with the ancient wisdom of effortlessness. Through the art of effortlessness, a foundation is built and a new approach to daily life is embodied—not laziness, self-absorption, or detachment, but the ability to be at ease and effort less within the parade of life's events.

Qigong Relaxation
The awareness of effortlessness

When life becomes stressful and you feel a bit separated from this ease, a return to the basics—in a qigong class, or in line at a store—will bring you right back in a moment, on a strong foundation and at ease with life as it is.

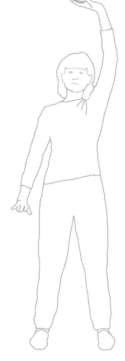

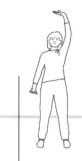

chapter 8

the art of
the qigong stance

THE QIGONG STANCE is the central element for all qigong exercise and meditation. This stance, crafted over centuries, ensures qigong's effect on the body's relationship to qi by improving qi flows through a process of increasing, refining, and balancing qi. Taking time to focus and learn these important steps will be more than rewarded with increased health, well-being, and sexual vitality. The stance simultaneously coordinates the proper ease of posture, deep breathing, sinking into the form as a relaxation, and training the mind in guiding the flows of qi. As these are correctly coordinated in the body, subtler components of qi and qigong are revealed. The stance provides the basic building blocks necessary to begin the art of qigong.

> ## Learner's Attitude
>
> **N**o matter how skilled at or new to qigong I am, I know nothing. I am here to learn.

Benefits of the Qigong Stance

Qi, like a stream of water, moves best when unobstructed. The various distortions of posture create corresponding distortions in the qi flows. Stagnation, speeding, crowding, and lethargic flows lead to the deterioration of life. The qigong stance promotes smooth, refined qi flows, the purveyors of good health and well-being. The recognition and integration of high-quality, highly available qi is the quest of qigong.

Regular practice of the qigong stance transforms personal posture from stressed to tranquil by exposing and resolving tension held within. Posture, as a rule, is neither experienced nor expressed as a means to develop a rapport with qi. Instead, our posture generally reflects simply a coping response to life. Stress shows itself throughout the carriage of the body, and these areas of stress distort qi flows. The qigong stance is the perfect antidote to the negative effects of body stress. The stance, crafted to perfection, achieves internal comfort, peace, and relaxation. It is in this state of inner tranquility that qi flourishes.

As you get better at relaxing within your body, your stress pockets will allow you to know your relaxed state more deeply. We need contrast for clarity.

The qigong stance can change your life—and you haven't even moved a muscle.

Awareness increases by creating internal tranquility. The basic guidelines of the qigong stance provide the tools to take this inner state of alert relaxation to ever more rewarding depths.

The commitment to developing a relaxed familiarity with this ancient stance affords many advantages:

- The lungs, diaphragm, and abdomen have room to breathe deeply and freely. Greater breath brings in more qi.
- The rooted quality of the stance creates a nurturing environment for inner strength.
- The sinking into the form relieves years of prolonged discomfort carried unnecessarily in the muscles and joints.

Tension areas previously not recognized will become very apparent. Breathe into the center of the problem. Sink the tension down toward the rooted feet. Relax into and within the form. As is typical of qigong's wisdom, the tool for the successful stance is effortlessness. Establish an intent to peruse your body in tranquil observation. Focus on an area of tension, and breathe, settling downward. As you feel the particular tension area melt and open into the downward sinking, affirm: "My body is relaxed, and I am fully alert to my breath." It is at this point of stable, rooted relaxation that the control over your state of being is manifested. The stance—prone, seated, or standing—is the position of choice for increasing vitality and well-being.

Qigong Attitude

Developing awareness

Releasing into the form

Practice

The stance is so subtle it can easily be integrated into any life action, event, or experience. This adaptable stance ensures a constant means of qi enhancement throughout the day. You can turn something as mundane and ordinary as waiting into an active participation in increasing health and vitality by training your mind to return to the simple touchstones:

Head light

Spine lifted

Shoulders sinking

Joints relaxed

Feet rooted

Settle into the structure of the form

The ease implicit in the stance is best supported by comfortable, loose-fitting clothing. Non-slip shoes or bare feet facilitate the rooted support. Remove anything even slightly restrictive—jewelry, watches, eyeglasses. Your goal is to completely free the blood, lymph, breath, and qi circulatory systems.

Qigong

Relaxing into and within the form of this process never ceases. The masters are still releasing ever deeper.

Stance

Feel as if you are a tree, a sequoia, rooted through your feet, roots extending down from the soles of your feet far into the Earth. Rooted, relaxed, and lifting upward, you are so relaxed and open it is as if the air and qi are breathing you.

As with all things practiced, the ease of the stance will become an integrated, unconscious part of your own personal movement sequences. Action, stance, action, stance. In qi language, this becomes: disperse energy, restore energy, disperse energy, restore energy.

The Standing Qigong Stance

Chest: Soft and relaxed (but not caved in), rising and falling easily with the breath

Abdomen: Soft, rolling easily with the breath, soft and rounded, not flat

Tongue: Resting gently on the roof of the mouth

The stance is tranquility and dynamic receptivity. It is this combination that makes the stance the centerpiece of qigong practice. The stance connects one qigong posture to another, forming the bridge between them. It allows the dan tian to get about its business of storing, cultivating, and refining qi for maximum benefit to body, mind, and spirit.

The basic stance guidelines that facilitate these advantages are simple and straightforward.

> **Breath**
>
> **W**hen doing the qigong stance, wear comfortable clothing. Particular attention should be paid to unrestricted breathing down the entire body.

Eyes: Softly open, vision emanating from deep within the head

Head: Lifted, elevating, moving easily on the neck

Spine: Long and opening, and perceived to be as strongly flexible as a rope; gently drawn upward like a sword smoothly drawn from its sheath

Shoulders: Hanging off the spine, relaxed, sinking down, but not rolling forward or drawn back

Joints: Elbows, fingers, knees, and toes relaxed and open, not locked

Feet: Fully on the ground, shoulders' width apart, toes relaxed

Throughout a sequence of postures, the stance is the center, returned to and departed from in every transition. This shift between posture and stance ensures that the body will respond with balance and grace. Grace of movement translates into a tranquil state of mind.

Each component of the stance has within it keys of awareness to open its value.

Neck and Head

Free the neck and bring qi to the brain. As the head gently lifts, the neck is free to release its considerable tension outward, downward, and upward. As these muscles lengthen and return to natural elasticity, the qi can nourish all of the elements of the head, most importantly the brain.

Chinese Instruction for the Stance

Quan Shen Fang Song: Whole body relaxed

Guan Jie Song Kai: Joints relax open

Xu Ling Ding Jing: Empty the neck, let energy reach the crown

Ding Tou Xuan: Suspend head

She Ding Shang E: Tongue reaches the roof of the mouth

Chen Jian Zhui Zhou: Sink the shoulders, drop the elbows

Zhong Zheng: Central and erect

Han Xiong Ba Bei: Sink the chest, lift the back

Song Kua: Relax the Kua (fold at juncture of thigh and torso)

Yong Yi, Bu Yong Li: Use intent, not force

Qi Chen Dan Tien: Qi sinks to the Dan Tien

—Kenneth S. Cohen, *The Way of Qigong*

Spine

The head is lifted upward. Light, it moves on the spine, elongating it. This sense of gentle elongation contributes to a new sense of flexibility. The head, spine, and neck create a line of continuity and stability throughout the stance. Your mind gently guides your head to lift and be light.

Joints

The joints are hinges in the body. Use your mind to conceive of each joint as a hinge. Rigid or tightly locked, they will not receive and transmit qi. Instead, the qi pools around the joints, creating stagnation.

When you release the joints, qi travels through your body from the relaxed, rooted toes up to the medulla at the top of the spine, and then to the head. Open each hinge. (If tension prevails in a specific area, move on. Return to it the next day and the next, and over time it, too, will loosen its hinge.) As each joint relaxes, the head is freer to relax on the neck and retain its lightness. Feel the line from the heels up through the spine and neck to the head. Let that line extend up through the top of the head (where the hair swirls on the very top, at the back). This lifts the head up without tilting the head backward or forward. Let your eyes relax back into your skull, and your sight will emanate from deep within your head.

Shoulders, Arms, and Fingers

Sink is the word for this area. The shoulders sink. The elbows release as a byproduct of the sinking shoulders. Tension will reverberate between these two areas, one creating stiffness within the other. As the shoulders sink and the elbow hinges open, the wrists expand and the fingers and thumbs show their openness by curling. And the shoulders continue to sink.

Spine and Back

The spine consists of a stack of vertebrae. Lifting the spine, by mentally pulling up the cord extending up from the head, lifts and opens the stacked vertebrae. It is from this flexible superhighway of nerves and qi that the stance moves. The spine is the core of the stance. Your head floats upward, your tailbone sinks down, and the spine moves freely and flexibly between the two. Your hips will naturally roll slightly under and in. This should be a natural process. Don't get a picture in your mind of how this should look and then mimic the picture. Let your body find its own point of equilibrium. All ease, no trying. Centered, stable, and naturally curved.

Let your chest sink. As your chest sinks, lift your back. The spine will free the movement (a sword lifting). In turn, the back will free the spine. This is an extension and a lifting of the spine. Sink the chest. Lift the back.

Hips

The home of the dan tian—qi's center in the body—is deep in the center of the pelvis. The hips provide the movement mechanism to liberate the dan tian from tension and poor use. Considered pivotal in the qi health of the body, the hips provide shelter and nurturing for the dan tian—by the nature of the body structure. As the hips free up from deep pelvic tension, the dan

Presence, Not Presenting

Posture is seldom an expression of the personal desire to receive qi. Instead, posture generally reflects the attempt, sometimes a labor-intensive effort, to hold oneself erect and unmoving. Often the posture has more presenting in it than quiet receptivity.

The qigong stance is the expression of the art of rooted ease and internal tranquility.

tian is freed to increase its function. The qigong movements and qi movement become sensitive to a newly found inner direction.

Are You Relaxed

What is the temperature of your hands? Qigong masters' hands are like warm, glowing suns. Their hands are actually so filled with qi that just shaking hands with them can be healing.

Mind

Qi follows the mind's direction. This is a most powerful statement, filled with profound meaning. All of qigong is a system designed to hone the mind's ability to direct the life of the body and spirit. The more you are focused, the more qi arrives to assist you in your mental pursuit. Qi will follow wherever you lead it and energize whatever your mind leads it to. Intent, awareness, and focus that are sloppy cannot assist anyone. Qigong stance strengthens intent and focus. Increased awareness then refines and disperses with wisdom the life-giving properties of the qi.

The Pelvis and the Dan Tian

The nourishment of the dan tian is the centerpiece of the qigong stance. This nourishment is provided by a technique of ultimate simplicity, *chen*, or "sink." Following the guidelines for the body's balance in the stance brings about the perfect environment for this final and very important step—as you lift, open, and soften to sink. Release downward, sink downward, let the breath deepen through the lungs to the solar plexus and into the pelvis.

Make no attempt to maintain a held-in, flat stomach. To nourish the dan tian, the abdominal wall moves like a wave on the sand, rolling out and back with rhythmic ease. Focus your intent on the very center of the pelvis.

As you move your mind to this area, between the hips and an inch and a half below the navel, deep in the pelvic center, a spot of warmth and aliveness will be revealed. This is the dan tian, the vessel of qi accumulation, refinement, and dispersal.

The dan tian is the vital center of all qi movement. The way to nurture it and support it in the accomplishment of its task is to sink—sink into the form of the stance and sink the breath deeper and deeper to find a warm union with the dan tian. The nourishment of the dan tian provides inner warmth, security, self-esteem, and self-empowerment. These components create an internal environment that allows you to experience confidence in spontaneous action.

Tongue

The placement of the tongue on the roof of the mouth joins together the two qi flows of the central meridian. This meridian runs from the perineum up the front and up the back. In the fetus, it is a constant circular flow. When the first sound comes at birth, the circular flow is broken into two flows. Putting the tongue on the roof of the mouth reestablishes the circular flow. This is a great contribution to balancing qi throughout the body. Many students develop the habit of always having the tongue at rest with the tip touching the roof of the mouth. It takes some practice, but it is well worth the effort.

The qualities of liberation associated with the qigong stance are experienced in these ways.

Presence: Increasing awareness of one's internal and external environment

Internal peace: Revealing and releasing unnecessary inner tension

Attentive ease: Incorporating effortlessness

Lively awareness: Being rooted

Well-being: Perfecting balance of Earth (di) qi and heavenly (tian) qi

Seated or Prone Qigong Stance

It is not possible for everyone to stand for a long period of time. In these situations the stance should be practiced either prone or seated. The guidelines remain the same. Don't relax too much. The prone or seated qigong stance is still a state of dynamic relaxation. Lift, open, breathe, and soften as if you were standing on your feet. Sink toward your feet, not toward the chair or bed. Press your feet against a flat surface. Resist getting drowsy. Dynamic relaxation means that, on the outside, you are unmoving—but you are filled with internal awareness.

Sequential Relaxation

The natural balance that occurs as a result of the stance is further enhanced by the space in which you practice qigong. Outside is great. Inside works too. An environment that encourages ease of movement through clean air and visual inspiration is best.

 When filled with qi, the body is like a tree branch filled with sap. It can bend and flow with the breeze, but it does not snap or lose its connection with the root.　　　　　—Kenneth S. Cohen, *The Way of Qigong*

These stances—prone, seated, standing—can be done in a developmental sequence: prone to seated, and seated to standing. Or one can choose one stance consistently and continuously. The determining factor is physical ability. Qigong will join you wherever you are.

The Prone Stance

Lie down on a comfortable, preferably firm surface. You are lying supported by the surface, but you are not limply relaxing onto the surface. This can be more easily achieved if you keep your eyes open, but the internal state is often easier to achieve with the eyes closed—your call. Using the surface as a support only, go through the qigong stance guidelines.

Become aware of your body. Maintain your position as if you were standing. Your feet can be pressed against a vertical surface for grounding. A tool for success is the expressed intent to "stand" on the vertical surface with ease and effortlessness: "My body is completely relaxed, and I am fully alert to and in my breath." Spine elongated, head light, joints relaxed.

Systematically travel through your body from the scalp down. Settle the scalp, the features of the jaw, the jaw, the chin. Settle the neck and throat down. The shoulders drop. Arms, elbows, and fingers relax and open. The settling continues through the torso. A releasing wave of supple breath encour-

---

Take a moment to gather your thoughts about what "stance" means to you. . . .

Take a stance.

I have my stance.

What is your stance?

The word usually implies a strong position, often one that is held against an external force of some sort. Except in qigong. Stance in qigong is dedicated to regulating the qi flow through stillness and attention, creating receptive relaxation.

Often we think of relaxation as a final step before sleep, a misty state of diffused awareness coupled with a slack body. In contrast, in qigong stance, relaxation is a state of heightened awareness combined with a surrendered release of tension throughout the body. Become familiar with this state of awareness while prone or seated. Then transfer that awareness to a standing stance of relaxed readiness.

ages the settling into your prone form. Your chest is soft; ribs and lungs lift and release; organs relax; the lower back opens through the hips; the thighs, knees, and calves release down; the feet are rooted—the bubbling spring is deepening and widening the roots into the Earth. You are relaxed and alert. Your breath moves in and out with a supple ease. Shift the focus from your lungs to your breath and the supple rise and fall of your abdomen. Allow your intent to rest on the emerging warmth of the dan tian.

Terminate if you get sleepy. Practice sustaining the prone stance for up to thirty minutes without experiencing drowsiness.

Once you feel completely comfortable with the prone stance, move to the seated stance, if you are able to do so.

The Seated Stance

Use a chair that is firm. Move away from the back so you support your torso, spine, and head yourself. Your legs should be uncrossed, your feet a shoulders' width apart and rooted to the ground. Keep your shoulders relaxed and open, arms folded at the elbow, hands in your lap, relaxed and open.

Initiate the qigong stance sequence:

Eyes are open or closed.

Light head floats upward.

Neck releases out and down.

Spine elongates up, like a flexible rope.

Chest is soft and sinking, and back lifts up and opens.

Hips open, pelvis relaxes.

Joints open and soften.

Feet are rooted, drawing the legs down, legs settling.

As the head rises, the joints open and you sink into the form, creating a state of lively relaxation, openness, and awareness. Repeat the relaxation sequence in the prone stance.

> ## Qigong
>
> It is not a matter of learning something new. It is releasing to return to a deep wisdom.

To learn the art of the qigong stance is to embrace the qi concept. Apply the relaxing sequentially, and release into the form. This restores the feeling of pleasurable ease associated with open acceptance of qi and its gifts. The qigong stance returns you to your own comfortable, easy relationship with yourself and allows the fountain of vitality to flow unobstructed through your body and soul.

Grounding Experiences

Become a mountain. Each step is like a silent, small earthquake. Elevate the head; your spine hangs like a flexible rope, and from the hips down you are planted.

Imagine sand is draining out of your shoulder joints. Your shoulders are sinking.

Imagine sand draining out of each vertebra of your spine, especially the tight and painful areas. Your spine is extending upward, a sword drawn from its sheath.

Your hip joints are leaking sand. Your hips become freer, more stable, and settle down into your legs.

Your feet are releasing sand through the bubbling well point. The roots into the earth are growing wide and deep as your body settles into the support the feet provide.

Return your stress to the earth:

The root is wide and deep.

 Sink down into the earth.

 Your head drifts upward.

 Your chest is soft.

 Your spine is supple.

 Settle into the form and release stress down.

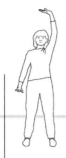

chapter 9
developing stability

I N ALL QIGONG PRACTICE, seeking the ground is essential. The definition of groundedness or rootedness is stability developed by maintaining a firm connection with the Earth. Rootedness creates strength and stability of the body, mind, emotions, and spirit. A well-rooted person has physical strength, mental focus, calm appropriate reactions, and the ability to nurture the soul with tranquility. The components creating rootedness are rooted feet, a well-settled center, and a graceful balance.

Rootedness demands a settling within the body. Tensions go in the opposite direction, pulling you up from Earth or simply holding tightly in place, but as you settle, these tensions will begin to merge into the settling-down feeling. A new experience of comfort will emerge. Instead of using tension incorrectly to maintain an erect posture, you will feel the release of relying on your body's own structure, which is perfectly evolved to accomplish just this task. You will allow the ground to support you and cease pulling away from rootedness through upward contraction and lifting. This accommodation to the structure's function allows your muscles to relax even more. The struggle to remain erect ends, and your muscles settle into natural elasticity. Your breath brings proper oxygenation. Qi

Find the bubbling well point to facilitate growing your roots. On the underside of your foot, notice the ball of the foot—one side connected to the toes and the other to the body of the foot. Running a hand over this lower connection, notice an indentation at the point where the ball curves upward.

This is a very important acupressure point for increasing the downward flow of the body. It is from the strength of this flow that the sensation of rootedness emerges. You can make these actual flows deep as well as wide. Simply press the tip of your finger or thumb into the point, apply pressure, and rotate counterclockwise.

settles into the dan tian. Since qi is very much like water, the coarse elements will settle toward the bottom, while the more refined, gentler qi rises above. In this way the undesirable qi of anger, jealousy, greed, fear, and the like, filters down, down, down and finally is released into the Earth. The refined qi clears the mind, refines the emotions, and the development of rootedness is now at hand.

Relax into the ground through your feet. Think of standing not on your feet, but instead in the ground.

Focusing Your Mind

The word root is wisely used. Picture a favorite tree. Qigong rootedness imitates that tree. Deep and wide roots, a solid trunk, light and moving branches and leaves. An invisible root springs downward from the foot. This root, flowing from the bubbling well, will provide the stability needed to accomplish qigong. The use of the mind to enhance this feeling is also a part of the initial training. Qi follows the direction of the mind, or in Chinese, *yi*. Your mind must first be able to guide qi, and rooting, with the bubbling well exercise, is a perfect beginning. The mind can visualize or command the qi flow leaving the bubbling well, flowing downward, wide and deep. Or the mind can concentrate on the bottom of the foot, creating heightened sensitivity, and feel the qi descending. All of these and more are varied styles of using the mind to direct qi. Any style that works for you is fine: visualize, command, sense, feel. All are equally successful from qi's perspective. Because your mind guides qi, it is important for the mental awareness to expand and practice focusing. The goal of qigong is to become ever more skilled at guiding qi. Leading qi to the bubbling well and getting familiar with mentally guiding qi are the first steps toward actually getting the qi to root into the ground. Now the qi goes beyond the feet, deep into the ground. This builds the roots. These roots, one from each foot, will become as real as any other part of the body. Qi becomes real, and the ability to communicate with the ground is born. This is true stability, qigong style.

Once the root is planted, the center becomes fuller. The ability to keep one's center will allow the qi to develop, increase, refine, and balance evenly. Center your mind on your dan tian. The roots are deep. Blend your mind into your body simply by thinking of the dan tian. Settle further into your body. The breath settles, the qi settles to the dan tian, and your roots are deep and wide. Notice that when the awareness of the dan tian is weakened through distraction, the qi is guided to the distraction (qi follows mind), and weakening occurs. As you develop the ability to focus your mind to root and guide qi to the dan tian through breath, settling, and focus, your mental and physical aspects become coordinated. This harmonizing facilitates guiding the qi throughout and beyond the body. Eventually this skill of nurturing the dan tian with breath and mind becomes the foundation for all thought, emotion, and action in your world. The qigong student is then never ungrounded, off-center, scattered, or distracted. Being centered and complete in each action becomes your way of life.

Balance is the natural outcome of rootedness and dan tian centering. It is the third aspect born from the merging of the two. Qigong balance is the balancing of the physical body and qi. The essential component for success is a balanced, tranquil mind guiding qi to rootedness and centering.

> Look at a tree. Think of the tree with its roots. Imagine how deep, wide, and complex the root structure is. Understand that the tree is borne upward from its roots. There is no separation between the roots and the trunk. Be as the tree borne upward from your roots.

Components of Rootedness

Tranquility

Ease

Sensitivity and awareness

Warmth

Life is made up of two intermingling flows of qi, Earth qi (di qi) and heaven qi (tian qi). These then flow into human qi and merge to create ren qi. The intent to learn through qigong's rooted, centered balance ensures the state of *Tian Rin He Yi*—Heaven and Human in Harmonious Unity.

Rootedness is initially learned and honed in the qigong stance. As the mind forms the habit of guiding qi and centering in the dan tian, skill develops. A point is reached when movement can be integrated into the form, and the rootedness and centering stay intact. "Form follows function" were the words Frank Lloyd Wright lived by. They are also the teaching of qigong masters. The form of the movement provides the function of the movement of qi. The way the arm is lifted or the leg moved is designed to create open, liberated pathways for qi to course through. The trained mind then guides the qi upward from the roots, from the dan tian, guiding the qi to the palms. The body is moved in a carefully crafted, ancient system to facilitate this qi flow. Muscles are relaxed, and a feeling of pushing starts through the relaxed arms. Elbows root the movement and are kept down, pointed toward the floor. With the elbows down, the forearms lift. The wrists are limp until the qi fills the wrists, strengthening them, and moves into the palms for the push. One flowing movement—rooted feet, centered dan tian, and in the case of arm movement, a grounding fork of the elbow.

Performing the qigong grounding exercise is not unlike being a traditional hunter, waiting for prey—quiet, in tune, blending in, invisible, waiting in alert relaxation for that moment of perfect timing to act decisively.

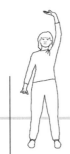

breath practice

BREATH and its fellow voyager, qi, are the reason for qigong. How qi's existence first became known will never be certain. Suffice it to say that as soon as qi was recognized as a vital component of breath, an ardent seeker began to pursue and devise ways to increase the personal advantages offered by this discovery. Survival was the taskmaster then. Having more qi enabled the hunters and protectors of children to be more effective. As life became more secure, the human relationship with qi assisted evolution by creating a high standard for achievement. High levels of qi set an example of what is possible in physical strength, emotional sensitivity, mental focus and clarity, and spiritual attunement. Qi's ability to assist with a current challenge and simultaneously create a vision of what else is possible has made it more valuable than gold. This easy availability of qi in the breath allows anyone to chart a course toward health and well-being.

Qigong Breath

With this generous abundance of qi available, the only challenge we have is our ability to breathe. Qigong teaches deep breathing. Deep breath differs from full breaths in the lungs alone. Although it is the most familiar style of breathing, simple lung breathing is actually quite inefficient in supplying the body with the nutrients of gas, blood, and qi that it craves. Society often creates an environment where breath is restricted. Stress—mental and emotional—as well as physical injury contribute to a type of breathing that is far shallower than is beneficial, a breath focused on simply inflating the lungs. Becoming acquainted with your own personal breath cycle is essential for well-being.

Stretch out, on your back if possible. Relax. Let the universe breathe you. Sink more and more deeply into your pattern of breathing. Notice:

- Is your abdomen rising and falling?
- Are your lungs extending down as well as out?

- Is your throat relaxed, and is your tongue touching the roof of your mouth?
- Are your lips soft, and is your jaw relaxed?

Feel comfort with the ease of your breath flow. Allow yourself time to become well aware of your breath's movement as you stretch out.

Move to a sitting position, allow the breath to breathe you, and notice any changes in your breathing pattern. Has the breath changed? Is the depth of breath the same? Are you as relaxed? If there are changes, where are they? Note any developments that restrict deep breath—that is, breath in which the abdomen and lower lungs are involved.

 The first six weeks require the greatest focus of will to carve time for breath regulation practice. If you remember to practice three times during the day, it will help both your practice and your life.

Now stand and once again notice changes in the pattern of breath. Are there any areas of restriction? Is the breath apt to be wide, expanding the lungs up and out only, rather than deep, down into the lower lobes of the lungs and into the abdomen? Make a few notes to yourself on the variations in your breath pattern. The areas of tension that became more obvious as the positions changed are ripe for you to open up with deepening breath and a feeling of settling into the area of tension. Become aware of your internally stressed or rigid areas. Soften them and allow the breath to move throughout your body. As you create this mental image, the mind directs the qi throughout the body as well. In some areas of stress—the shoulders, hips, and lower back are a few—this may be the first time in a very long time that qi has flowed in and out without stagnating. This, in turn, provides a feeling of pleasant well-being. It can be useful to keep a brief record of your progress in using breath regulation and qi intake to create a new order within your body.

Unless otherwise indicated, it is best to do qigong breathing through your nose, with your jaw relaxed, and your lips full-feeling and lightly closed or slightly parted. The tip of your tongue should touch the roof of your mouth. Your eyes should be open, gazing in a relaxed manner at a point ahead. Feel your vision coming from points deep within your head—not from the surface of the eyeball, but from deep within.

Natural Breath

This is the path of natural ease for the natural breath—the first qigong breath. This means exactly what the name implies. This is the breath of the child, the sleeping adult, and the experienced meditator. The breath flows into the nostrils and falls to the lungs, the diaphragm contracts downward, and the abdomen rounds out to a still point of fullness. The breath flows out, the diaphragm relaxes and rises upward, and the abdomen comes inward, reaching a still point of emptiness.

This is a breath filled with natural ease. As nature's way of providing breath and qi in abundance to the body, natural breath will adapt perfectly to the body's various needs. Resting, exerting, getting ready for action, and deep relaxation to increase awareness all make different oxygen qi demands upon the body.

It is not necessary to stay in a daily state of heightened awareness about your breath's various adaptive styles. Simply work with the now-familiar qigong stance and gentle breath regulation. As this becomes more and more familiar, and then comfortable, breathing in general will improve, twenty-four/seven.

Aspire to a breath that is slow and steady, and a rate of inhaling and exhaling that is nourishing and unhurried. This encourages a breath with a long, even quality. The qi will sink into the depths of the dan tian. A delicate quality enters the breath at this point. The mind suspends its fervent activity, its concerns about the past and future, and fills with tranquility. Indeed, true tranquility is the state of perfect attainment. Qigong opens the path to tranquility, and from this delightful state the gifts of qigong spill forth.

Breath is described as a twofold (inhale/exhale) process, when in actuality it is a fourfold process, with each component having an equal and vast influence.

Inhalation: This involves relaxing and opening the body to receive the breath and qi.

Qigong practice that is done not only in practice time, but also at other points during the day, increases your receptivity. The qigong masters believe that God—Love, Wu Chi, the Universe (it is called many names)—surrounds us continually, embodies us through qi, and is always available to lead us to our true nature. Only our inability to be receptive interferes with our awareness of this constant support. Qigong done at any time, in its entirety or in snippets, reinforces this connection. It is the all-purpose anti-stressor.

Transition at fullness: Here the breath turns (you can feel it) and prepares for the exhalation. It is a balance point of inner stillness that nibbles away at anxiety.

Exhalation: This is the release as the breath flows back to the universe. Releasing and letting go facilitate an increasing ease with life, as the need to control and micromanage diminishes.

Transition in emptiness: Now comes a moment of calm, encouraging wise reflection and acceptance.

When you practice qigong during the day, it actually feels as if time is slowing down. This is one characteristic of connection to omnipresence.

There is great good that can come from feeling the transition points keenly. It is from feeling these brief but consistent encounters that we can derive a calmer approach to life, a better sense of our own timing, and a clearer understanding of self and responsibility. These transition moments act like brief gateways that allow a flash of expanded perception to occur. In advanced states of breath exploration and regulation, much tranquil awareness is given to these transition points.

Six Qualities of Breath

Slow – Man

Long – Chang

Deep – Shen

Fine – Xi

Even – Jun

Tranquil – Jing

—Kenneth S. Cohen,
    The Way of Qigong

Reverse Breath

Since we are dealing with an age-old, sophisticated Chinese tradition, there are naturally hundreds of forms of breath regulation. These make up the variations in qigong, which are legion. The breath techniques are variations on themes, and one of the themes is natural breath. Another is reverse breath. Reverse breath, in this context, is to be used as a supplemental breath technique to support deeper access to natural breathing.

In reverse breath, the abdomen's actions are exactly the opposite of those in the natural breath. When you inhale, the abdomen pulls in. When you exhale, the abdomen releases out. The entire focus is, once again, on the breath, the dan tian, and the qi settling into the dan tian. This approach to breath is best achieved in three steps, keeping in mind several points:

- The breath is slow, never quick.
- The body is relaxed, except for the specified action of the abdomen.
- The techniques are used for brief periods of time, to support the regulation of the natural breath.

There are three methods that are appropriate for this form of learning. (Advanced breath regulation should always be done under the guidance of a qualified qigong instructor.)

1. Keep your focus on the contracting and releasing of the abdomen as the breath slides in and out.
2. Through focus you will note that, when you inhale, the qi is elevated from the dan tian in the pelvis. There are actually three dan tian energy centers. The dan tian in the pelvis, in the solar plexus, and at the third eye, or the point between the eyebrows. The reverse breath enables a shifting of the accumulating qi from the center dan tian to the solar plexus dan tian. As your skill and interest increase, pursue the form of qigong breath that focuses on and nourishes these energy centers. Each center affects perception. The pelvic dan tian creates a grounded, relaxed, well-energized pelvis to center and charge the body. The solar plexus dan tian nourishes quick action and split-second timing. The brow dan tian is the site of the ability to extend one's perceptions through and beyond the physical. The second and third dan tian cannot develop the fullness of their potential without the pelvic dan tian being fully functional. For this reason, use the reverse breath to open up and support your entrance into the full, complete, and very satisfying natural breath that sinks to the pelvic dan tian.
3. The reverse breath done briefly will break up the breath restrictions that stress has built up in the diaphragm. The reverse breath is an excellent way to become present very quickly. The reverse breath can bring you into an alert state if you're inappropriately sleepy. It is excellent for strengthening the abdominal muscles and therefore the lower back. These results can be achieved in up to, but no more than, three minutes of practice.

Reverse breath is a useful tool to create a specific outcome in specific circumstances. It is natural breath, however, that holds the qigong treasure chest of reward.

Other Types of Breathing

These are the identified forms of breath regulation that have been generated through the venerated tradition of qigong:

- Natural Breathing: As we discussed, this is the regular breath pattern that is maintained unassisted by the body.
- Cleansing Breath: This energizes the nose and the mouth. Inhale through the nose, exhale through the mouth. This is useful if you feel unwell. Focus your mind on an area of discomfort and breathe natural, easy breaths through the nose and into the identified area. Then exhale through the mouth, letting discomfort flow out with the breath. This is also a useful technique for releasing limiting emotions. Inhale through your nose, identifying the breath as earmarked to find that emotion (remember, qi follows mind—a mind-boggling premise if you really focus on what it means), then exhale the offending emotion through the mouth. You will experience relief, although maintenance may be required for a while. The emphasis is on the ease and depth of the directed inhalation and then the committed expulsion of the breath. When you sigh, your body is organically accessing the cleansing breath. When you feel a sigh coming on, open your mouth, and the sigh will accomplish more.
- Toning Breath: Inhale through your mouth and exhale through your nose. This is a fine breath first thing in the morning, with the window flung open, taking in good big gulps of qi for the day. It improves overall energy and inspires circulation. This breath will be manifested naturally when lifting something heavy, diving under water, or getting mentally ready to do an unwelcome task.
- Alternate Breath: Common in yoga classes, this breath alternates the flows between the nostrils: inhaling through one and then exhaling the breath through the other, inhaling through the same nostril that just exhaled and then exhaling through the opposite nostril. The index finger and thumb of one hand can open and close the nostrils as needed to inhale and exhale correctly.

  This breath calms disrupted emotions and can relieve head and neck pain. Locate the pain, direct your mind to the area, and exhale the pain with the breath. The technique can be made more effective by matching the side the pain is on with the nostril on the same side. Temporal headache on the right side of the head? Use reverse breath with the cleansing focus on the right nostril, switch to the left, and then return the focus to

Often when we build up our breath for exertion, or to hold it, we take great big breaths, filling the lungs to the tippy-top. Experiment with this. Fill up to the top and measure the time you can hold the breath or the distance of the sprint you can run. Now breathe deeply, but in a relaxed and natural way. Fill the lungs about three-quarters full, starting in the abdomen, and now see how you do. Generally the body does better with the three-quarters full breath because relaxed muscles provide better endurance.

the right. As the irritated qi dissipates, the pain will subside.

- Deep Breath: This is an aspect of natural breath. It is the spontaneous deep breath that accompanies relief from great stress, a beautiful view, good air, the sight of a longed-for person. The body shows delight by taking a huge, easy, deep breath. This can be facilitated by stretching your arms up and wide while thinking about what you are grateful for. It can be used to disengage from worry and to encourage a good night's rest.

- Tortoise Breath: This is the breath of the master—slow—three to six breaths per minute (the average number of breaths per minute is sixteen). The Tortoise Breath is not forced by the practitioner. It just simply comes with mastery.

In each of the previously mentioned breathing techniques, the emphasis will shift from the movement of the lungs to the movement, contraction, and expansion that surrounds the dan tian. When the entire mind is lost in focus on the dan tian, the breathing occurs without your conscious involvement. This is the sure secret to success with qigong breath work. When focusing on the lungs, you're not dealing with the bottom line, but when you move awareness from the respiratory breath to the movement of the dan tian, you end up where you should be. Your breath, qigong breath, and all your awareness are focused on nourishing the dan tian.

Breath Awareness

A tour through these various ancient techniques clearly demonstrates the profound skill with which the qigong masters explored the variations on breath that naturally occur in the body. Breath became a tool for better health, a means to emotional balance, a bridge to the sharpening of spiritual perception, and the essence of the master's craft for improving every aspect of human behavior and action. As a beginner, you will find it useful to add to your journal of breath awareness some notations on how your body naturally responds to breath. These are useful, self-probing, awareness-increasing questions:

To someone noticing you doing a breath exercise, it would look as if you're just repeating the same exercise over and over again. Outwardly, qigong looks repetitive, but to the practitioner it is a kaleidoscope-like experience that is simply framed by the guidelines of the exercise. To know qigong, one must be within the frame.

- Where is my body tight and restricted?
- Can I direct my breath into the area and bring in more space?
- Is my pelvis warm and supple?
- Can I feel the "pouch" of the dan tian when I focus on it?
- As my lungs expand, am I settling into the dan tian?
- Do my shoulders seem to move apart a bit as I inhale?
- What is the area under my collarbone doing as I inhale? As I exhale?
- Is my back reacting to the expansion of the inhalation? To the release of the exhalation?

Your entire body actually responds to the breath. When you inhale, your legs stretch, your hips expand, your spine lengthens, your shoulders widen, your arms and hands lengthen out slightly, your neck opens, your head lifts, and the plates on the bony structure of your skull move apart slightly. This all reverses when you exhale. With so much going on structurally, it is a small step to understanding how the organs open and aerate, the diaphragm and lungs lift and open, the circulatory system gets more oxygenated, skin tone improves, the brain receives more qi, and all of life is looking good. Deep qigong breathing is a natural ticket to general overall improvement.

It is useful to remember that qigong breath was born from the natural curiosity produced when someone observed the body's natural breath rhythms and then tried to understand them better through personal exploration. The forms and systems of breath regulation are fascinating and open up vistas to be explored—and you are your own best environment for exploration and self-awareness.

Embrace natural, spontaneous breath. Resist the temptation to depend on a system or the teacher so deeply that you distance yourself from your own rhythm, your own timing. Your breath is your timing, and the absorption of qi is a mix especially designed by you for you. Revel in the breath. Open your body, mind, and heart to the natural elixir. When you are completely attuned with your own breathing, you will notice a time when the breath becomes so slender that it seems as if you might not be breathing at all, and yet there is no sense of deprivation of oxygen or comfort. This is a state of protracted effortlessness when you and the breath are at a point of equanimity. Ease and quietude fill the experience and provide a balance point where the two transition points can be explored by just settling into them as they roll through. This state is most easily achieved in passive qigong—still, without yin, dynamic within yourself—but can become a part of qigong movement if practiced consistently over time. These are indeed memorable movements. It is a blissful state of harmony with breath and qi. Typically these times first occur only during qigong practice, but over time they can be extended into daily life. You are fully present, completely at ease, and profoundly balanced by the breath, qi, and dan tian.

> Integrating qigong into life in bite-sized pieces is an effective way to progress. Like all of the Eastern disciplines, it deepens in meaning and rewards over time. Practice is the traditional and ideal way to evolve in qigong, but integrating it into your everyday life brings the benefit level up another notch.

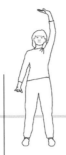

chapter 11
qigong meditation

HERE ARE THREE LEVELS of awareness—waking, sleeping, and meditating—and the function of any form of meditation is to seek and find that third level of awareness. Meditative states can be reached in the rhythm of long walks, watching a river flow, gazing at clouds, or in the relaxed and tranquil state of mind when settling into the rhythm of familiar physical chores. We now have a culture where these natural areas of life are being squeezed away, and with them goes the ability to nurture our third state of awareness within the context of our everyday life rhythms.

There are 2 styles of Qigong Meditation:

☞ ru jing, to enter tranquility
☞ cun si, the art of healing visualizations

Each skill is useful to learn—Ru jing for satisfying our essential need for inner quiet; Cun si for learning how to direct qi through the mind.

Enter the meditative techniques from the East. It is the frustration of not achieving this satisfaction that creates obsessive thought and anxiety. Qigong meditation encourages the release of persistent and annoying thoughts as we become more familiar with reshaping a life with more satisfaction, and less frustration, woven into it. Meditation returns right timing to the process of daily life so that our responses to life situations are satisfying and comfortable.

There are two basic forms of qigong meditation. The first is *Ru jing*, which teaches us how to be dynamically involved with the inner world of qi and tranquility. Tranquility in this form of meditation allows the mind to release into a void of non-thought and in so doing arrive at the state of satisfaction inherent in being. Over time a myriad of techniques have developed to facilitate tranquil being. Keep in mind that these systems are meant to serve as an entrance point to tranquility. They cease to be useful when they become demanding, so that the technique or the system becomes the goal, instead of the means to the goal of tranquility. Don't lose yourself in technique and forget to just breathe, be, and allow all else to be. Satisfaction is the key, breath is the door, and tranquility is the discovered space.

The other basic form of qigong meditation involves training the mind. This second form is best incorporated after the mind has relearned how to release unnecessary thought. This second qigong meditative style takes a more pliable, receptive mind and begins to introduce specific mind-guiding exercises to retrain the mind to create life-enhancing thought. The value of this is enormous, because qi follows the mind—anywhere and everywhere—and there it infuses its aliveness. An undisciplined mind energizes aspects, situations, emotional responses, and fears that hamper efforts to construct a life that is well loved and lived. This qigong meditation, *Cuu si*, is the mind-developing craft of using visualization, focused concentration, and specific feeling states to teach the mind to direct qi in well-thought-out, decisive, and life-enhancing ways. Empowered positive thinking is the result as thoughts are constructed to replace ways of thinking that are habitual, repetitive, and generally negative.

Visualization is used to create sharpened awareness. This awareness, somewhat like a sharp surgeon's knife, is inserted into the pattern of an outdated or negative thought pattern and, with precision, the released thought is replaced with the new thought pattern that has been decided on. This is not like using the sand-draining exercises for stress reduction. Those are indeed visualizations, or perceptions, but they work within existing conditions to bring relief and satisfaction. Instead, qigong Cuu si takes visual images, new ways of perceiving, and focused concentration, and lays in a new pattern. For example, let's say your back hurts. The sand-draining exercises can give you release from the pain, and the movement of qigong can keep it from returning. But if you stop doing them, the pain returns. Qigong Cuu si, instead, creates a clear visual pattern of your back as healthy and permanently free of pain. The skill of the technique is the way the new thought pattern is inserted to replace the old thought pattern that is supported—of course, unconsciously—by the back.

These qigong meditation techniques are dynamic and result-oriented. One can certainly attain a typical meditative state as a result of the visualization, but that is not the goal of the effort. Ru jing (tranquility) and Cuu si (visual guidance of the mind) both create healing. Both utilize qi. One supports the other.

One cannot overemphasize the impact of qi that follows the mind's thoughts and then manifests what is there. Poor self-esteem can create a perception or life-view that validates the feeling of worthlessness. If qi does follow the mind,

Some of Meditation's Benefits:

☞ Improves qi flow

☞ Purifies the meridians

☞ Clears the brain

☞ Calms and clarifies the mind

☞ Clears excess emotion

☞ Strengthens the immune system

☞ Slows down stress induced aging

☞ Improves the ability to focus

☞ Increases inner and outer harmony

☞ Facilities deep easy breath improving oxygenation

☞ Improves connection to the omnipresent

☞ Improves ones ability to affect health positively and directly

☞ Enhances compassion and equanimity

as the Chinese masters heartily believed, then meditation can just as powerfully project life energy into desired life attitudes or events. Using whichever technique—imagination, visualization, or focus—feels most natural, you can redirect self-esteem issues, instead of being crippled by them. Imagine, visualize, or focus and concentrate on another reaction to a situation. Make it feel real. Over time this leads to remarkable and truly lasting changes, and low self-esteem becomes self-confidence.

These techniques can be applied to any life event. Health responds to deep belief. Go deeply enough into a belief, and a physical change can be created as a powerful, although not the only, influence on health and well-being. It cannot cure everything, but it is powerful enough that it is worth every moment invested in learning the qigong meditation.

How can you know if a health or well-being issue is mutable and therefore alterable, or if it's cast in stone, unless you pursue it to your greatest depths? It is in those depths that great liberation is found.

Focusing on one's own healing is a central piece of Cuu si. The wellspring of Cuu si is the care and nurturing of one another and nature. Prayer is now being demonstrated as an enormously useful tool to assist others to greater levels of health or loving support in a deteriorating situation. Prayer is another example of the way qi follows the guidance of the mind, then contributes.

Qigong visualization is a "done-deal" approach. The body—your own or another's—is visualized, experienced, and fully concentrated on as whole and healed, and filled with the nourishing warmth of qi. The qigong approach to visualization can be combined with the more familiar approach to healing body and emotions through visualization. This more familiar approach works with the situation as it is. Lower back pain? The back is visualized as releasing its pain. A variety of images can be used here—draining sand, a warm sun melting the pain, sweeping the pain up into a dustpan with a broom and throwing it away. Each person will have a unique creative idea, usually emerging easily from the unconscious. The pain recedes under the focus of the mental visualization. At this point the qigong done-deal style can be utilized. Now a picture of the entire body free of pain, moving easily, flexible and healthy, is created visually. As this vision is held, the qi moves to create the image. The qi, now freed up and balanced through qigong movement, carries its vision throughout the body. The body responds by accelerating its healing process.

Ill health is often not a simple fix, and many forms of treatment may be appropriate. Qigong visualization meditations are a tremendous support to any healing modality. Sometimes seen as acceptable because it is harmless, it instead proves the great intrinsic value of mind focus, concentration, and clear visualization.

Meditation Techniques

These meditations are best done with the guidance of a qualified qigong teacher. One meditation a day is a full experience. Practiced regularly, one consistent meditation can have an obvious effect. Learn to do one well, rather than skipping around from one to another. The techniques use many different approaches, so it is not hard to find one that fits well. Settle into it as you settle into the form in the qigong stance. After you have grown accustomed to one, it is useful to branch out and utilize the variety to assist you in life.

This is the advantage of learning such ancient movements and meditations. They have been applied to many, many states of disharmony. Successful outcomes were recorded and the technique used and reused century after century. With each generation, its success has deepened as it improved with the passage of time. Qigong masters have taken the art of visualization to a highly developed level. The ability to visualize the body as perfectly healed, whole, and filled with youthful vitality became, with practice, the ability to meld the body with the visualization and become it, in a moment. This was then taken a step further by developing the ability to move the mind-qi connection into any part of the body, where, in this environment of intensely intimate self-contact, it was very useful for self-healings and self-redirecting of conscious-ness. The understanding of the energetic workings of the body became increasingly clear. Both the evolving techniques and the outcomes were metic-ulously recorded. Unfortunately, most of this astonishing wisdom is waiting to be translated and published in the Western world. But start with the basic meditations outlined in this chapter. This was where these men of ancient times started as well. The qi is speeding up now, coursing more quickly than it was during their time. This speeds up the entire process of life, but it also makes it possible to reach into these realms of self-awareness more quickly. Thus, the following exercises, simple as they are, will take you far.

Meditation Technique: Tranquility

This meditation technique provides an entry point to inner tranquility. Even when you're feeling your most stressed and frenetic, you carry in your deepest nature an attunement with tranquility. The outer world of Earth is filled with tranquility, as is the universe. Your breath can create a bridge for you. Medita-tive breath will connect you to the web of tranquility. Life is still life, but you will become more filled with peace and inner reflection.

Let this be easy for you. Don't set goals on how it will be or what you should be accomplishing. This is like relaxing at the end of a busy and satisfying day. The work is done; the day is over, and you are disengaging from the day's busi-ness, letting the day close down behind you. If you have things to do later or the next day that intrude on your thoughts, write them down. Remind your mind that these things don't need to be remembered or resolved now. This is downtime.

Sit comfortably, back straight, neck and head supported, if possible. Your body should be relaxed.

Let the breath breathe into you and out of you as you relax into this source of life flowing in and out. Place your tongue tip against the roof of your mouth. Breathe in and say to yourself, "I am." When the breath peaks of its own accord, say "calm," and when the breath turns into the exhalation, finish with, "...and relaxed." Settle into the words combined to the breath and the rhythm of the breath/word sequence. The words and the breath combine to form an intent which gently filters into the cells of your body. Each rhythmic wave of breath and word carries profound tranquility. As the words flow with breath, let your mind rest upon the breath, a bit like a sheet settling down on a mattress as the bed is freshly made. Feel the rhythm of your breath. As you do nothing but settle into the state being created, you might hear your heartbeat. Or you may hear a very quiet roar—this is the nervous system. Light, sound, and color may all be a part of this. Or there may be nothing but the breath and the words. Either way, you will be creating a larger space for tranquility to reside within by removing stress to where it belongs, on the outside.

Take time each day to gently close your eyes. Attune to your breath. Align words with the breath, and take a minute or more to return to the natural and needed third state of awareness.

Walking, sleeping and meditating: Each one needs the other two to function at maximum productivity.

The breath/qi is where life begins and ends; don't underestimate its influence on the process in between. Meditation can make you more cognizant of the breath/qi's wealth of resources.

Meditation Technique: Mind Guidance

This meditation uses the regulation or guidance of the mind to improve overall health: All breath is inhaled through the nose, exhaled through the mouth, and done three to five minutes per organ.

- Choose the organ you want to start with.
- Bring your awareness to that organ.
- Inhale in the color associated with that organ: exquisite, light-filled color.
- Exhale. A darker color exits when you exhale, dark and heavy.

Organ	Color	Sound
Liver	Green	Shuuu
Heart	Red	Ho
Spleen	Yellow	Hoooo
Lungs	White	See-ahh
Kidneys	Black	Chrrooee

- Repeat the inhalation with the color.
- The organ permeates with light.
- Exhale, and the darkened colors release and exit.
- Inhale again the exquisite color.
- Gaze into the organ and see it filled with color. The color rests within the organ, suffusing it with exquisite radiance.
- Exhale normally. More dark color may or may not emerge.
- Inhale again into the glowing organ.
- Breathe normally and naturally.
- Gaze at the beautiful organ.

Move on to the next organ and repeat the process exactly. Different color, same exquisite radiance. Repeat with each organ.

It is very useful when feeling ill to bring healing to the affected organ. This exercise will also balance the emotions and improve mental clarity.

To enhance the organ breathing:

- As you exhale, say the sound that is associated with the organ, in a loud whisper.

It is best to do all five organs in sequence. Where you start in the sequence is your call.

These are but a few techniques passed on to us by qigong's dedicated lineage. If one or two appeal to you more than the others, begin there. Over time, your capacity to engage with a wider variety will increase. This occurs as a result of learning ever more about guiding qi with the breath and mind. Free up any assumptions you may have gathered regarding meditation. Simply experience what is suggested by following the steps and then making the technique yours. Each one of these meditations has the capacity to give you a gentle, sturdy support and a fascinating understanding of the value of expanding awareness.

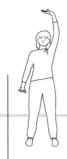

chapter 12

awakening your mental powers

THE MIND simply has the power to create, and like any great power source, it needs guidance and boundaries to reach its full potential.

Medicine is finding that the mind has a tremendous influence on the body. This is not to deny the importance of other factors such as environmental toxins, nutritionally compromised food, genetic time clocks, and high-stress, low-yield lifestyles. Still, the dominating influence on health and well-being, or lack of it, is the mind. Regulating and gaining mastery over nonproductive aspects of the mind, then, becomes a matter of good health.

We're all aware of unproductive states of mind. A few include:

- A drifting mind floating aimlessly from one thing to another
- A very focused mind running like a plowshare through soil
- A flighty mind, hopping from subject to subject
- An expansive, information-gathering mind that is unable to focus

Qigong does not revere analysis over imagination or problem solving over fantasy. They are all equal in the eyes of mind regulation. Each offers another form of guiding thought toward creativity. Each can become too consuming and needs the balance of the other styles. The ultimate in thought is to bring it present and ground it.

In and of itself, each mental pattern is fine. The problem develops in the tendency to habituate. As one mode of mental pattern becomes more familiar, it lends itself to habit, and an overuse of one style of problem solving develops. It is this repetition that causes the problem. Habituation is the most negative state in life. It is the antithesis of qi freshness. Qigong provides an environment where the mind lets go, and in this release, it learns to become more effective. Habits of mind movement are adjusted to create an environment in which mind can begin to understand its amazing potential.

Perfecting the Thought of No-Thought

Qigong masters believe that the value of the qigong session rests on the answer to one question: Was thought stopped? This is the challenge of qigong.

Learning the sequential movements is fun. Coordinating breath and movement brings a sense of security and release. Stopping the flow of the mind is a different challenge. We need the mind to remember the sequential movements and the breath coordination. How can the mind, then, be taught to stop? The mind doesn't really stop. It is being trained to achieve something different—a unification of the mind with the movement and breath. This is the state of "thought of no-thought." The mind guides the body. This brings a sense of firmness within the relaxation. The mind learns to ride the breath; the mind learns to sense the qi, and then the mind learns to guide the qi. Mind, thus engaged, becomes completely separate from the influence of life. Mind is not in the past. Mind is not in the future. Nor is it constructing a fantasy or an idea. When "thought of no-thought" occurs, your mind can glimpse calm. A steadiness emerges. Groundedness is enhanced. The emotions balance. Qigong can now be pursued for what it offers. This achievement requires commitment, exertion, and perseverance. The mind gives up its compulsive attachment to problem solving, ideas, and ramping up of emotions. It finds it is capable of much more. It will seek to experience a level of awareness where it can pursue the business of life *and* be filled with peace and light. The mind's need to expand reaches into a higher potential of relaxation and new exploration.

It is at this point that the mind approaches its initial glimpse of the potential for unification. The mind settles into the body, flows with the qi, seeks, feels, senses the qi, and communicates directly with the organs. This communication reaches the point where qigong practitioners are able to practice the art of internal vision—*nei shi gongfu*.

It is at this level that the mind explores internal realms. At this level, you can sense the elements of the body through the mind's awareness. You can become more effective in color breathing by seeing the colors associated with the organs (see chapter 11). It is from this point of self-awareness that the five-element theory (see chapter 3) becomes a living reality.

This level of mind perception is available to all practitioners, each in her or his own time. Resist setting your goal on this type of achievement. Set your focused concentration on your "no thought." Your mind and breath settle into the dan tian. In this way you are practicing *yi shou dan*

tian—the mind staying on the dan tian. The student and the master are the same here. The point of attention is the fountain of qi. The love of staying attuned to qi's nourishment is a life commitment. The dan tian roots the qi, and the rooted qi then follows the guidance of the mind.

Qigong Mind

Qi is a flow, like water, and therefore it cannot be pushed with effort, but it can be led or guided. Mind is blended with breath to achieve this. For instance, say you want to take a step and raise your arm. You inhale into the leg and arm from the dan tian, send qi to the areas, and when the qi has brought liveliness to the muscle, you move. Would the movement be possible without this preamble? Of course, but you wouldn't be as strong or peaceful. The mind always leads with intent, and the body follows. When the qigong practitioner can sense qi, then the guiding of the qi with the mind develops a new level of potency. Learn the truth of qi through the experience of qigong, and then take this new awareness and apply it.

Qi is an invisible world that we get to live in.

Initially, the application is focused on one's self. The entire qigong commitment is concentration on one's self: getting the movement right, weaving in the breath, taking beginning steps in managing the mind so it will yield to direction. The mind is given to problem solving. Put the mind in an environment where the immediate problems are greatly diminished, and you have a chance of getting its attention and guiding it. This is an environment of simplicity and balance that provides a shield of grace from the cares of the outer world. Not a world to escape into, but a world that is satisfying. The element of satisfaction

Nature's way is the wisest influence in health and well-being. Qigong doesn't impose its will on nature. Instead, qigong provides a way to heighten one's sensitivity to nature and guide qi in accordance with her rules and will.

diminishes the mind's need to solve problems in the present. The task simplifies. Draw the compulsively active parts of the mind back from the past and future and into what is happening now. A simple and freeing movement is occurring in the present moment: qigong class!

The first focus is breath, mind, and movement, but as skill increases, the ability and desire to use the mind effectively in expanding circumstances emerges. Consciously or unconsciously, the movement to improve the life around you to a more satisfying level permeates the will. The tools learned in the qigong practice become applicable to larger and larger environments. There are well-documented steps to developing these skills.

The Steps

Mind and Body

This is where qigong takes you first. You must have awareness of yourself in relationship to qi and the wisdom it carries. "To thine own self by true" can only work if we know ourselves. This awareness of the self is achieved by a sense of being found through groundedness. What groundedness teaches is a direct, uncluttered experience of your body, simple and straightforward. This is sought and found by establishing a direct relationship with Earth.

When the mind has become unregulated, there is no steady groundedness in being and Earth. Instead, there is more a flitting back and forth between body and the travels of the mind. Here, there, everywhere, ideas, fantasies, and solutions fill our attention. Our ability to have a full and happy life is enormously affected by our ability to ground ourselves in our body's beingness. Settle into the breath, and the body is nurtured. Natural survival anxieties abate. The mind, less burdened by the body's anxieties, is taught the first step.

The ancient qigong masters preferred to draw qi from the breath and the pure morning dew than to eat large amounts of food.

Mind and breath travel as companions. A breath that helps train the mind consists of:

Exhalation: The connection, the communication. The mind travels on the exhalation to make a contact.

Base of the Exhalation: The dissolving. The connection is released, and a space occurs.

Inhalation: The mind waits as the breath flows in.

Peak of the Inhalation: The breath turns. The mind is in the turn.

Exhalation: The mind travels on the exhalation, and contact is made.

To Rest the Mind: Rest in the dan tian, grounded.

Since we are working in a world where time and space are not simply physical, mind can travel on a short exhalation to the tip of the nose or to the far reaches of the universe. Mind can go wherever qi flows, which is everywhere.

As you learn this, you will do qigong, breathe, ground, think, and then remind yourself to think of breath, think of no-thought. Sometimes thought floats here, sometimes there. When this occurs, give your thoughts little grounded feet. The now grounded thoughts join your body through the breath. Qigong groundedness supports your thoughts' sense of well-being. Without the little feet, thoughts become floating, flitting. Now there is a home ground. Like a true home, this one offers a thriving environment to return to. Your home is your grounded body. Breath and mind return to it and enrich it. This dynamic is reenacted in the qigong sequences. Center and ground, move from the center into movement, return to center, move from center into movement, tethered and unfettered.

Mind and Life

As you progress through qigong, it will become clear that qi is the practice of mind regulation. This generates a stronger intent

Linking Mind and Breath

It is important to breathe in through the nose and then gradually lengthen the breaths down to the dan tian. The breath may feel as if it is thinning with the descent.

For complete breaths, bring your attention to the dan tian. When the dan tian is moving like a gentle bellows, the amount of breath in the lungs will be satisfying. Generally, this is about 70 to 80 percent of full lung capacity. Breathing into the lungs and taking deep breaths stresses the muscles, and they can't take in as much oxygen.

to practice with precision and attention. Very quickly, attachment—that natural desire to possess that which has personal value—asserts itself. Attachment promotes the body's survival anxieties. The body's need to be assured of its ongoing survival is all-consuming. When focused on the qigong experience, the attachment suffocates the very experience being sought. The essential ground through the body has been sought and found. Moving with the qi and finding the essence of life within the movement evokes enormous satisfaction . . . and a great tendency to cling to the form to regain the experience. This couples with the fear that it won't return again. Anxiety develops around doing the form correctly to get the longed-for experience. Comparison with a previous experience occurs. The practice becomes a struggle.

A search for the predictable, the desire to recreate something from the past, a hope for future fulfillment—this is the mind struggling to find balance between the tangible body and the dissolving qi. This balance is a new relationship for awareness. Contact the experience and let it go. You are there in the movement, present and in mindful connection, mindful awareness. Then you let go, dissolve. Then back to present mindfulness—grounded, dissolving.

Holding onto qi contradicts its nature. Qi can be directed, but not captured, contained, or controlled. Qi is spontaneity. Qi is fresh. Qi flows. Qi is omnipresent. To attach to qi and attempt control has only one outcome: qigong becomes just another task and responsibility in life, something else on the list to get through. The gift of qi so exquisitely sensed before will no longer be available. Resentment is the next logical result.

Finding freedom from this state of attachment is an ongoing process. Here are a few clues for successfully moving through and beyond attachment:

- Focus your mind on that which you recognize as what you are desiring. Then let go of the object and release. Move on. Your breath can help you with this.
  - Inhale.
  - The breath turns.
  - Exhale, release.
  - Dissolve, let go, and move on.
- Survival anxiety can be approached with: I have survived. I am here. Breath, qi, and me. I am here, and that is enough.
- An acceptance that we are all on loan to one another. The universe calls back the loan when it is ready. Exhale, release, accept. Inhale, turn, exhale. This particular realization helps encourage greater presence and appreciation for what is now, who is now, and a recognition of the effect

of omnipresence in our lives.

- By accepting these recognitions, your qigong practice and the awareness attained from it become applicable to life. Directly address your survival and attachment concerns in the midst of qigong.
  - Inhale: I am here. Address the survival concerns.
  - The breath turns.
  - Exhale: Let go and flow out
  - Dissolve, dissolve.

This is extremely helpful because it puts qigong and your life experience in the same place. They are becoming inseparable from each other. As a result, life-giving qi and its wisdom manifest themselves continuously in the mind. This union brings clarity of mind, an upgrade in intelligence, and an improvement in the skill of living. Many realizations will emerge. Dominant will be an understanding of touching life. Be the presence of life and go. You will learn to be in the moment, like the exhalation—to go but not leave. Just be present. Give up analysis, reinforcing, because they interfere with the qi flow, in and of life, and are therefore no longer as desirable. Qigong reaches out (exhale), returns to a grounded center (inhale). Your thoughts reach out and return to a grounded body. This is the light, free, and efficient movement in life.

Mind and Effort

So where does effort come into all this? The difference between worldly effort and qigong effort is like that between forcing a door and slipping in a key that turns the tumblers easily. Exertion is an essential component for learning qigong. Effort is counter to all of qigong. Qigong is not deliberate, but precise. It is not heavy-handed, but light. A series of qigong movements progresses in an unstoppable flow filled with contained dignity and grace, slow and steady yet filled with light and playfulness. Qigong is too important to be taken seriously.

There is a big difference between heavy-handedness and light application. Take advantage of a most natural, instinctive flow. Bring the mind back to the breath. Take it away from the intensity it has become attached to. Draw the mind back from its zealous wanderings. Cease to let it make strong claims on what qi should be doing. Just return it to the breath.

This is not a series of sequential steps. It is a gentle reunion. The return of mind to the grounded body through breath brings a moment of clarity, a moment when exertion comes from within and is therefore devoid of effort. This clarity becomes the lens through which life is engaged. Life is now perceived with a variety of opportunities. Choice of responses expands. Opportunity is chosen, and response is chosen, with mind, breath, and body in union, and presence to express self. It is a moment like being in love. In that instant, clarity and interaction become the rhythm that unifies everything with perfect timing. There is no effort. The mind in union with body, breath, and qi—clear perception is the outcome, exquisite timing is the reward, and omnipresent love is the realization.

Mind in Mind

Mind moves in sequential steps. Designed to take in information and create, it moves through events one experience at a time. Multitasking is not an example of mind doing three things at once, but just sequencing faster. Mind integrated into breath and movement develops an intellectual alertness and presence. It is unlike the observational process that merely watches, disengaged. Qigong mind carries the qualities of a refined mind arousing to itself. Awakened, the mind now lives with the body, with the survival concerns, with desire, and with itself. Mind is now able to be present and everywhere.

The sense of experience expands with the joyous awareness that each of us bears complete personal responsibility for the quality of life lived and expressed. Each life is unique and never again to be repeated. You can do nothing to tear yourself from the fabric of life. You cannot throw it or yourself away. Mind in mind recognizes this state of pure aliveness. You experience a complete picture with nothing absent; then you let go and move on. Another perfect picture, nothing absent. Let go, move on. There is no repetition. Each thing happens once. It all happens in sequence.

Mind will go wherever it is sent. It is fun to experiment with this and useful for your qigong practice. You are making your mind facile, learning to direct it, and having fun. Each one of these exercises is a dimension of mind guidance:

1. Color Breathing. For good skin, imagine you have a light pink cloud surrounding you. As you inhale, you bring the cloud into and under your skin. Exhale through your mouth. Repeat ten times.

2. Saying Hello to an Animal. Animals are telepathic, and they experience communication in the moment it occurs. A flock of birds will change direction simultaneously. They are in the moment of the communication. It is like this with all animals. They are the mind in the oneness of life.

   Imagine you have a probe or a finger of qi extending from your forehead to touch an animal of your choice. Fill this mental extension with nurturing appreciation for the animal, for its beauty, its softness, its inspiration. With your thoughts, appreciate it. Make a picture in your mind to match your words. Animals will respond instantaneously to your "hello." Their experience with other human beings will affect their willingness to interact. Keep at it. You will have some wonderful experiences.

3. Qi Comfort. You see or are with a person you want to extend comfort to. Using your mind, direct your qi to come out of you on both sides, like two arms. Extend your qi arms around the person, leaving some open space in back. The person will be more relaxed and comforted.

4. Your Own Space. Take a string about nine to twelve feet long and make a circle on the floor. Step into the center, sit down, and say, "This is my space. I am completely responsible for the quality of self I express from this space. This is my qi space. Mine, and mine alone." Imagine the string actually marks out a qi membrane. An arm's length away, it surrounds you completely. Imagine you are drawing this membrane right up against your skin, making your qi field small. Return it to its egg form. Now imagine that you are extending it out to make full, boundaried contact with the walls of the room. Or send it out to make contact with a tree—complete surface contact between you and every bump, leaf, and branch of the tree. Draw it back to its egg form. Now bring the qi boundary up against something else in nature—a creek, fish, flower, tree, or the like—and make the boundary porous. Merge your qi field with nature. Lighten the pores on the boundary and return it to the egg shape. (It is not recommended to merge with human beings.)

5. For Pain. Next time you hurt yourself, "brush" the qi above the wound, not touching it. Brush up and then brush down. See which movement helps relieve the pain. You are stopping the qi from piling up at the wound and causing irritation. A qigong master will be able to drop mind into the wound and heal it quickly by delivering high-quality, healing qi as it is needed.

A t the end of a mind-guiding sequence, you may feel a bit different. You are in an altered state. You can alter your mind back to a more familiar state — another guiding of the mind. This time sense your skin, the soles of your feet. Take a deep breath and relax it out. Finally, do something very familiar and ordinary: Put on your shoes, brush your teeth, take a shower, call a friend. The familiarity of the action will ground you.

None of these is a classic qigong mind exercise, but each holds a world of experience in it. They can become clear illustrations of the tremendous range of talent the mind carries when directing qi. They will also help you understand how guiding the mind works best for you. This knowledge can be applied to your mind-regulating exercises as you venture into qigong.

qigong sequences

HOOSING from among the fabulous variety of qigong forms illustrates the intrinsic and flexible value of qigong. There are forms to help with every aspect of life and struggle. One is as valuable as the next. Some are older, some more revered, others newer but nonetheless used a great deal. In *Qigong Basics* you will be introduced to three different forms that service three different arenas of human concern. Enjoy experimenting. Quite possibly you will find that you have a deeper accord with one than with the others. Learn the whole sequence or take a snippet. Learn it, embody it, settle into it, and develop ease with the sequential movement of your choice.

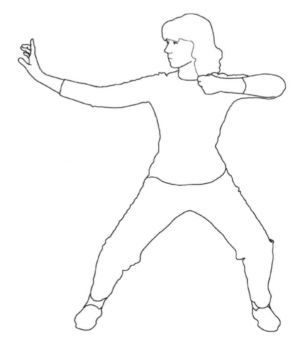

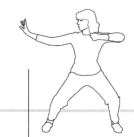

chapter 13
shaolin si qigong

THIS FORM OF QIGONG, Shaolin Si, comes from the qigong practices of the venerated Shao-lin monastery. First a Buddhist
temple, it later became the home of all martial arts. Located
in the Songshan Mountains of China, fifty miles from Zhengzhou, it is the pro-
vincial capital of the Henan Province. Known primarily in the West as *the*
training ground for martial arts, it is also one of China's oldest and most important Buddhist shrines.

Established as a Buddhist temple in 495 during the Northern Wei dynasty,
it was not until the mid-500s that it became a center for martial arts. This transition occurred partially because of the location of the temple. The location
developed into a strategic area, and the invasions, wars, and rebellions created
the need for self-protection. The second reason was the arrival of the Buddhist
monk Da Mo in 520. He arrived at the temple having trekked through the
Himalayan Mountains into China. As mentioned in chapter 1, he offended the
current emperor (Da Mo was unimpressed by the emperor's understanding of
Buddhism—which consisted largely of having monasteries built), so he left the
court, seeking an environment closer to the true search for inner enlightenment. He arrived at the temple during a time when the monks were in poor
physical condition. Their condition disturbed him, because it interfered with
the effectiveness of their meditations. He took a ten-year break to meditate
alone, and returned to the monastery with the first two forms of qigong and
martial arts to teach to the monks and help them improve their strength and
health. These forms were *Xi Sui Jing*, brain and marrow washing, and *Yi Ji Jing*,
muscle and tendon change. The monks flourished as they became stronger,
and their meditations and search for enlightenment strengthened.

The timing was such that the monk/warrior emerged when most needed
for China. In the Tang dynasty (618–906), thirteen trained Shaolin monks saved
the emperor, Li Shimin. From that moment on, the dynasty blessed the temple
with lands, wealth, and permission to continue refining qigong and the martial

arts. This imperial protection continued on into the Ming Dynasty—1368 to 1644—when the temple housed over three thousand monk warriors in constant, disciplined training. Qigong, martial arts, herbal medicine, and the guiding of qi were all utilized to create a peak of achievement for combat.

They were frequently called upon to assist in the emperor's ongoing battles. The monk warrior of this time set the standard of excellence in Chinese culture. A balance of martial art and qigong skill was sought through poetry, meditation, and reverence for nature.

A reversal of fortune occurred in the Qing dynasty, 1644–1911, when martial arts were declared forbidden. Concerned for the loss of their long-held protected status, the monks took qigong and the martial arts to the people. Training was motivated by a new need for assistance against the warring forces. The process of teaching these two, now vastly complex, movements was necessarily simplified. Training had to be sped up, and many intricacies in the form were lost, as well as the extraordinary skill that can only come after years of practice and discipline. Training techniques gained over a thousand years were lost, but the potential to arrive at these states of skill still remains.

The Shao-lin Temple has been damaged many times, most seriously in 1930 when a forty-day fire destroyed almost all of the temple's classical literature and records, then again in the 1970s by a band of Red Guard during China's Cultural Revolution. The Shao-lin Temple exists today and covers ten thousand acres. There are over three hundred ancient stone inscriptions, large and beautiful murals in the Eastern Halls, and 232 pagodas. The pagodas are shrines, tombs of celebrated Shao-lin monk-warriors.

Shaolin Si (Cosmos) qigong is a health art through which we experience what is pure and perfect in ourselves and express our gratitude for what we consciously receive and choose in our lives. We realize our interconnectedness with the larger world, and we have the opportunity to give back into our outer lives. Our inner world and outer world meet. Although it is a basic form of qigong, it is a profound exercise for attaining and maintaining health. This is the simplest version of the basic theme.

Preparation

In stand-ready position, the feet are close together, as comfortably as possible, connecting with the earth through the bubbling wells. The hands are relaxed at the sides, with the palms facing toward the back at an angle, body upright, though relaxed. Chest is soft, shoulders relaxed. The crown of the head is open toward heaven. We are the expression of the qi from heaven and the qi from the earth.

Breathing is relaxed, slow, calm, and continuous. The breath is the bridge between body and mind, calming the mind and the heart. We clear our mind of any thoughts, and we empty our hearts of any emotions. We create a quiet space within ourselves. We develop a "one-pointed mind," a mind that could lead the qi wherever it should go. We prepare ourselves to be conscious in all our qigong processes. We need to be fully mindful of the energies we connect to in each movement. We recognize that life has only one purpose, and that is to create life. We give life the space to perform this task through this simple qigong exercise. We smile from the heart.

Body of Exercise

First Section

Grounding and Centering

From stand-ready position, move into the Horse stance: Bend your knees slightly, with your weight on the right foot, lift your left foot and step to the left, in line with the right foot, coming down on your toes and then lowering your left heel. Shift your weight to 50 percent on each foot. The toes of both feet should be in line and facing directly forward, feet as wide apart as the shoulders. Keep your knees slightly bent, your weight sinking into the earth through your feet, your tailbone facing down to the earth, while your body remains relaxed. Keep your chest as loose as possible, your shoulders slightly rounded and relaxed. Focus forward (Figure 13-1). Follow the breath in through your nose and out through your mouth throughout the whole sequence, relaxing your stomach muscles as

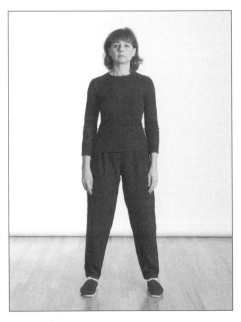

Figure 13-1

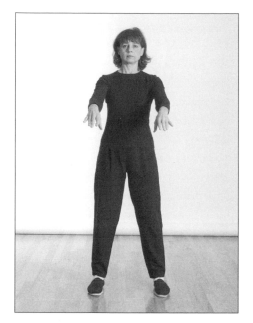

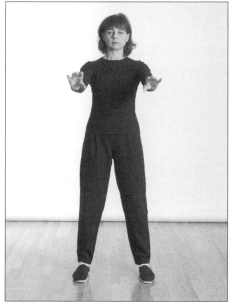

Figure 13-2   Figure 13-3

you inhale. Remain in this position until a state of relaxation and calm is achieved.

The traditional "Horse" stance is used for many forms of qigong. The stance allows for a firm, stable, and flexible base (legs). The head is held as if suspended from heaven. This posture allows qi from heaven, in the head, and qi of the Earth, in the sacrum, to flow freely.

Lift both hands up in front, with the elbows pointing down, the wrists relaxed and "leading" the hands up to shoulder height, while the hands remain a shoulders' width apart. Your knees should extend slightly. Inhale. (Figure 13-2.)

Drop your hands, with the wrists leading, to nearly waist height, while sinking slightly in the knees. Exhale. (Figure 13-3.)

These easy movements are called Grounding and Centering, as we lead the qi from the Earth through the bubbling wells and to the dan tian, the storehouse of qi in our bodies. As we exhale, we expel stale qi through the palms of the hands and the breath exhaled through the mouth.

Connecting with Source

Start on the right side and follow through for all the movements in the whole sequence. Move your right hand forward and upward, wrist leading, eyes

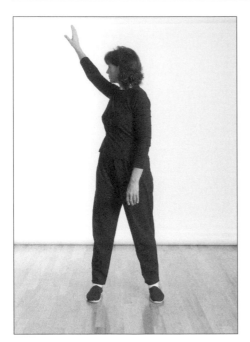
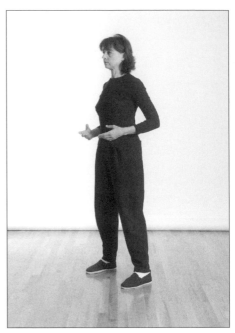

Figure 13-4   Figure 13-5

following the movement, to above your shoulder. Inhale.

Turn your waist, let your arm drop behind you, outstretched with the elbow relaxed and the palm facing down—the hand is stretched outward from the forearm. It makes a circle to the back and down to the side. Exhale, inhale, and exhale. (Figure 13-4.)

Your weight shifts to the left leg as your waist turns and your arm starts dropping toward the back. The weight changes to the center at the end of the second breath. The whole movement follows three breaths.

Repeat to the left, and alternate left and right for a total of three times with each arm.

We stretch out and up, our fingers and our whole being connecting with the source. The mental image we hold is that of connecting with perfection, that which is pure and true in ourselves.

Connecting with That Which Empowers Our Recognition of Source

Remain in the Horse stance. Draw your elbows back, while your hands rise on both sides, with the palms facing inward at an angle (Figure 13-5).

Inhale.

Create a large circle with your hands and arms in front of your chest.

Exhale, inhale, and exhale.

Turn your palms toward your body, facing your chest, and bring them closer, to three inches from your chest. Inhale.

Turn your palms down and lower your hands, pausing at the dan tian, and turn your palms towards the dan tian (see Figure 13-1). Lower your hands to your sides. Exhale.

Repeat this movement three times.

Here we honor acquired qi. We embrace and draw in that which is available to us in abundance—what we eat, drink and breathe. This empowers the "blueprint," the true design or "truth" of ourselves.

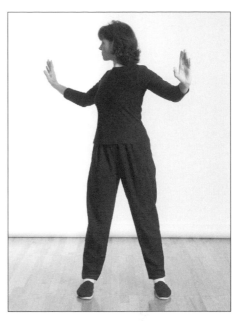

Figure 13-6

Connecting the Inner with the Outer Universe

Remain in the Horse stance. Turn to the right and extend your arms outward to the right and left. Face your palms forward, with your thumbs on top. Turn your head to face the right hand. Inhale and exhale. (Figure 13-6.)

Lift your hands slightly, drop your elbows (hands will withdraw a few inches), and re-extend your hands outward, with your fingers pointing away. Inhale and exhale.

Repeat this movement, now looking toward your left hand. Inhale and exhale. Repeat the movement for the third time facing the right (back) hand. Turn your body to face forward, dropping your hands. Inhale and exhale.

Repeat this sequence to the left.

We have received much from life, and in gratitude we offer life back to the universe. We mature in our relationship with the world around us. We accept our interdependence with the universe.

Connector between First and Second Sections

With the following movements we increase our defensive qi, particularly between the elbow and the fingertips.

In Horse stance, shift your weight to your left foot, and turn your right foot

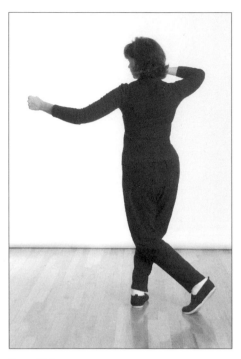

Figure 13-7

on the ball 45 degrees to the right. At the same time, lift your right hand to shoulder height, with the palm facing down. Inhale.

Step on your right heel, toes facing 90 degrees from your starting position, weight still on your left foot, with left knee bent. During this movement the right hand forms a fist facing down. Turn on your right heel, so your toes are 180 degrees from your starting position, and transfer your weight to your right foot. Turn on the ball of your left foot, bending your knee to "fit into" the back of your right knee. During this turn, while shifting your weight from your left to right foot, draw your right fist back to opposite your right ear. Simultaneously, form a fist with your left hand and punch forward, so that your fist lands to the right, 90 degrees from the starting position. Your head should be turned toward your left fist, and your torso at 45 degrees from the direction of the left fist. Your body should remain upright, with your eyes focused toward your left fist. Exhale. (Figure 13-7.)

Lower your left ankle, shift your weight to the left while turning your left fist to face you. Inhale.

Turn on the heel of your right foot, turn your right fist to face up (elbows are bent and facing down), turn your right foot to the original position, drawing your elbows back, with your fists facing up and resting on your hips, and your weight 50 percent on each foot. Exhale.

Repeat to the left, starting with opening your left hand, and stretch to the left, palm facing down, while shifting your weight to the right.

At the end, open your fists, make a circle with your hands, palm to palm, facing your body. Inhale.

Bring your palms to your chest and turn them down, letting them sink down to the center of your body and drop to your sides, while you shift your weight to the right, and step to the right with your left foot (stand-ready position). Exhale.

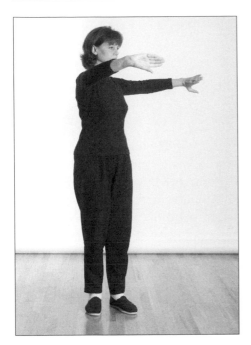

Figure 13-8

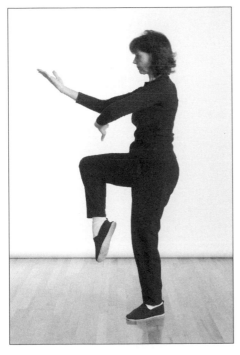

Figure 13-9

Second Section

Floating Eagle

In stand-ready position, turn your left foot out 45 degrees and turn your body to the same angle. Touch your left and right wrists together, right hand under left, palms facing at an angle toward the body. Lift your hands up and out to make a circle across your chest, palms now facing downward. Inhale. Slide your hands apart, drawing your elbows back, maintaining a circle, with your palms facing away from your body at an angle (Figure 13-8). Turn your waist in to the right, facing 45 degrees from the starting position. Exhale.

Turn your right hand over with the fingers leading down and the palm facing toward your body, while your knees sink down. As your hand passes your right hip, the palm facing up, start lifting your body up, bringing your right hand up and over the back of the left hand, fingers leading, right palm facing your body. As you raise your body, put your weight on your left foot (at 45 degrees). Lift the right knee, toes pointing down and knee slightly out at an angle. The right hand ends in front of your right eye, palm up at an angle, as the knee ends in the lifting position. The left palm faces away from your body at an angle; your right elbow is over the back of your left hand, and both hands are in front of the right side of the chest. Throughout the movement, maintain the focus on your right hand. Inhale. (Figure 13-9.)

Extending the Inner Universe into the Outer Universe

Step to the left with your right foot, coming down on the heel. Simultaneously bring your right hand toward your right ear. The toes of the right foot point forward, and the weight is on the right, with the left foot lifted onto the ball and both knees bent. Inhale.

Turn to the left, 90 degrees from the starting position, on the ball of your left foot, shifting 70–80 percent of your weight onto your right foot. Simultaneously, push your right hand forward, to end with the palm facing away at shoulder height, and draw your left hand back to the side, palm facing down. Exhale. (Figure 13-10.)

Circle your left foot around, and step into the Horse stance. Facing forward, bring your hands to circle in front of your chest. Your weight should be evenly distributed. Inhale and exhale.

Shifting your weight to the left, turn 45 degrees on the ball of your right foot, while turning your left palm up and your right palm down. Your hands remain in a circle away from your body. Inhale. (Figure 13-11.)

Step down on your right heel and repeat the same movement to the right, while extending the left hand forward. Exhale.

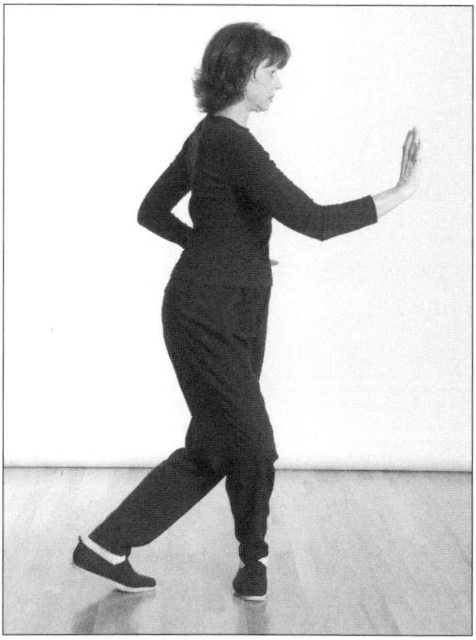

Bring your left foot around into the Horse stance, now facing to the back, away from the starting position, with your arms in a circle. Inhale and exhale. Shift your weight to the left, turning on the ball of your right foot, step down on the heel of your right foot, and turn to the forward position by bringing your left foot around. Your arms remain in a circle. Inhale and exhale.

Drop your hands to your sides, then lift your arms up and out to the side, palms up, until your palms meet above your head. Inhale. (Figure 13-12.)

Figure 13-10

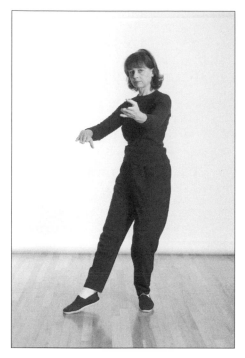

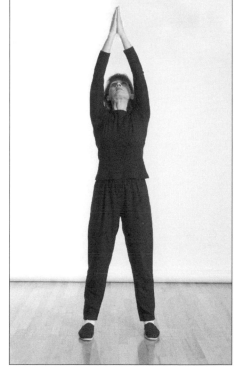

Figure 13-11 (above)

Figure 13-12 (right)

Bring your hands down, palms together in prayer fashion, then let them separate and fall naturally to your sides. Exhale, inhale, and exhale.

Shift your weight to the right and step right with your left foot, assuming the stand-ready position. Inhale and exhale.

During these seamless movements, we integrate with the energetic world around us. We are more than just one. We, and everything around us, are a unity. We extend what we are outward, taking on the power of the entire living universe.

Closing

Quietly relax, enjoying the fresh qi that you have accumulated and expelled into the world. With a quiet mind we trust in the healing ability of the body and allow our bodies to use the freshly acquired qi to heal us, throughout our bodies. This position could last for many minutes. Accumulate the qi at the dan tian by focusing on the dan tian.

Shake your hands and feet, or walk around briskly.

Our aim with these simple movements is to align ourselves with the truth of who we are. In doing so, we move into a state of wellness and integrity, or internal balance. We choose harmony and abundance with joy and gratitude in our hearts.

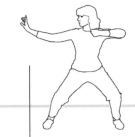

chapter 14

eight pieces
of brocade

EIGHT PIECES OF BROCADE is another form of qigong rich with
its own history. One story of the Eight Brocades' history is
this. Marshal Yue Fei molded it from another, longer form in
the mid-1100s. As mentioned in chapter 3, his concern was for the health of his
men, warriors who were under constant pressure to fight. The Song Dynasty
(960–1279) was a difficult time in Chinese history. Many wars with northern
nomads, as well as poor economics due to widespread corruption, resulted in
debilitating malnourishment and frequent starvation. Marshal Yue Fei, still
treasured in the memory of the people of China, was born in this era, but was
not of it. Like many young men of his time, he had a childhood filled with
turmoil and poverty. But when he was a teenager, his inherently noble qualities drew the attention of influential people, who contributed to his upbring-
ing, adding to the solid foundation his mother had given him. At nineteen he
entered the army and very rapidly rose within the ranks, becoming a general
by the age of twenty-six. As a general he was concerned for the ultimate success of his troops. As a previously impoverished person himself, he understood
his men's physical limits. He insisted that they be trained in martial arts as a
part of basic boot camp. This training proved essential for many men. Both
those who joined freely and those who were conscripted were often given a
weapon and sent to battle immediately, with no training. The martial arts
training produced good soldiers who had gratifying successes. He developed
the Eight Brocades as a support for his men's physical, mental, emotional, and
spiritual balance. Yue Fei was betrayed and killed by jealous and corrupt politi-
cians, but his Brocades have passed through the generations of the Chinese
people side by side with his revered history. He is known today as "Yue, the
righteous and respectable warrior."

The eight hundred fifty-year-old Eight Brocades form of qigong has inevita-

Jet Lag

If you are having trouble getting to sleep or waking up, the Eight Brocades can help adjust your body to the time zone. Sleep comes more easily, and in the morning you are more alert.

bly morphed into many variations. But, as with all of qigong, the most important element is not the form itself, but the theory, guidelines, and principles that cement all of qigong to its simple root. *Ba duan jin* translates to "Eight Pieces of Silk Brocade," a series of eight sequential movements that is easy to remember and graceful to watch and do. Marshal Yue Fei's well-conceived form is the essence of qigong simplicity and effectiveness. Repetition of these forms has bestowed long life on warriors, common people, and sages alike.

The Eight Brocades easily fits into a health regime. It can be the body of the workout or an effective warmup before a more strenuous workout. The decision about how to incorporate it is yours.

The Eight Brocades is an intriguing movement because it works specifically with balancing the basic meridian system within the body. This is why, in its

If you know that one of these systems is a bit weak or a possible trouble spot, then start the Eight Brocades during the two-hour period when that particular system is being nourished by qi. Each one has its time and takes its turn. The meridians are ordered into yin-yang partners.

Time	Meridian		Yin/Yang
7:00 a.m.–9:00 a.m.	Stomach	>	Yang
9:00 a.m.–11:00 a.m.	Spleen		Yin
11:00 a.m.–1:00 p.m.	Heart	>	Yin
1:00 p.m.–3:00 p.m.	Small intestine		Yang
3:00 p.m.–5:00 p.m.	Bladder	>	Yang
5:00 p.m.–7:00 p.m.	Kidney		Yin
7:00 p.m.–9:00 p.m.	Pericardium	>	Yin
9:00 p.m.–11:00 p.m.	Triple warmer		Yang
11:00 p.m.–1:00 a.m.	Gall bladder	>	Yang
1:00 a.m.–3:00 a.m.	Liver		Yin
3:00 a.m. – 5:00 a.m.	Lung	>	Yin
5:00 a.m. – 7:00 a.m.	Large intestine		Yang

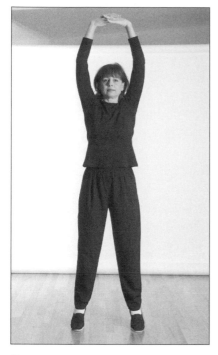

Figure 14-1: Position 1

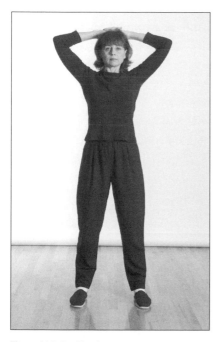

Figure 14-2: Position 2

simplicity, it is so effective in a wide variety of situations. If you are upset, it will calm you down. If your energy level is low, it will give you some spark. It is great for jet lag, a problem of the meridians lining up with a new sun zone. The reason it is so helpful in a wide variety of situations is simple—it restores balance.

There are many variations on the Eight Brocades. This one is based on Ken Cohen's excellent book *The Way of Qigong*.

Eight Brocades

First Sequence
This series balances the:
- Triple warmer meridian
- Pericardium meridian
- Destructive influences: stressful and disappointing human relationships
- Positive influences: acceptance, release

Inhale:
Move your feet a shoulders' width apart.
Bring your arms up and over your head.
Interlace your fingers above your head, palms up.
Rise up on your toes. (Figure 14-1.)

Exhale:
Return to flat feet.
Bring your interlaced fingers to the crown of your head. (Figure 14-2.)

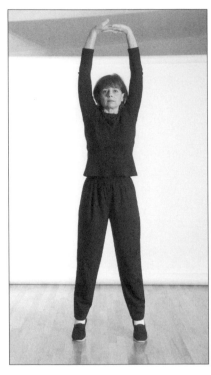

Figure 14-3: Position 3

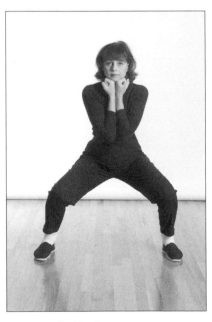

Figure 14-4: Position 4

Inhale:

Lift your arms upward.

Rise up on your toes.

Turn your palms upward. (Figure 14-3.)

Repeat the entire first sequence two to three times.

Second Sequence

This series balances the:

- Lung meridian
- Large intestine meridian
- Destructive influences: anxiety, unexpressed grief
- Positive influences: integration, integrity

Exhale:

Take a wide stance, with your knees comfortably bent.

(Go no deeper than thighs parallel to the floor, and keep your spine erect and up to avoid collapse in the pelvis.)

Make fists.

Roll your arms to bring your fists in at chest height.

Touch the backs of your hands together.

Tuck your chin under. (Figure 14-4.)

Inhale:

Bring your right fist to your right shoulder, with the right elbow extended and the right arm parallel to the floor.

Simultaneously:

Open your left hand.

Extend your left arm to the left, with the palm flat up and out. (Figure 14-5.)

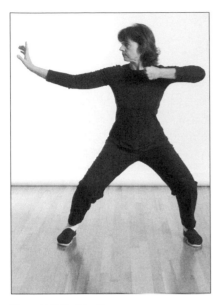

Figure 14-5: Position 5

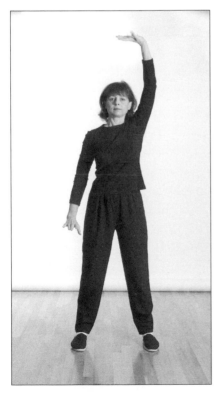

Figure 14-6: Position 6

Make fists of both hands, and return to the previous position.

Repeat the entire second sequence on alternate sides, two to three times each.

Third Sequence

This series balances the:

- Stomach meridian
- Spleen meridian
- Destructive influences: self-absorption, obsession
- Positive influences: trust in self, trust in life.

Inhale:

Stand with your feet a shoulders' width apart.

Lift up your left arm.

Bring your left hand to the crown of your head, palm up.

Your right arm is bent by your side.

Bring your right hand to your rib cage, palm down.

Push the two hands away from each other—left up to heaven, right down to Earth. (Figure 14-6.)

Exhale:

Circle your arms out to the sides to reverse the sequence.

Your head and eyes are forward, with a relaxed gaze.

Repeat the entire third sequence two to three times on both sides.

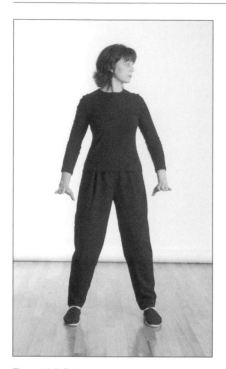

Figure 14-7: Position 7

Fourth Sequence

This series balances the:

- Gate between the head and body, relaxing the shoulders and neck, which improves spinal strength and cerebral circulation.

Breathe naturally:

Drop your arms to the side.

Press the heel of your palms toward the floor, letting the palms and fingers lift up.

Turn your head slowly and easily from side to side.

Keep your chin level.

Let your eyes gaze unfocused, looking from deep within your head. (Figure 14-4.)

Repeat the entire fourth sequence two to three times on each side.

Fifth Sequence

This series balances the:

- Heart meridian
- Small intestine meridian
- Destructive influence: shock, excessive joy
- Positive influence: creating balance and order

Take a wide but, of course, comfortable stance. Place your hands on your hips, thumbs to the back, fingers on thighs. Your body is going to swing easily and gracefully from side to side in this way. (Figure 14-8.)

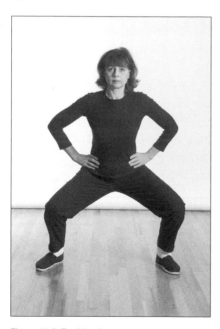

Figure 14-8: Position 8

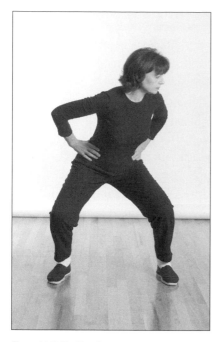

Figure 14-9: Position 9

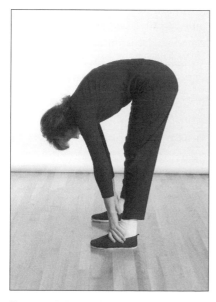

Figure 14-10: Position 10

Exhale:

Feet and bubbling well grounded, slowly swing your waist over either thigh, and bend toward the thigh.

With your body bent back straight, swing to the other thigh. (Figure 14-9.)

Inhale:

Easily and with no effort, straighten your back.

Return to center position.

Repeat the entire fifth sequence on both sides two to three times.

Sixth Sequence

This series balances the:

- Central meridian
- Upper and lower halves of the body, drawing in qi as the muscles at the back of the body relax
- Destructive influence: holding back
- Positive influence: sharing oneself with grace and self-acceptance

Exhale:

Stand comfortably, with your hands on your bottom.

Bend from your waist.

Slide your hands, palms in, down the backs of your legs.

Relax into a stretch.

Release the spine and let it lengthen. (Figure 14-10.)

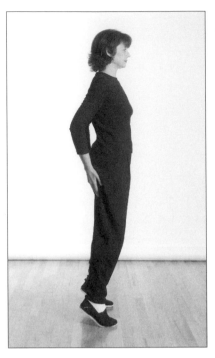

Figure 14-11: Position 11

Inhale:

Imagine planting a seed in the base of your spine, and let the growing sprout roll you to a standing position.

Slide your palms up along up the backs of your legs, following the sprout.

Bring your hands back to your bottom.

Rise up on your toes (peak of inhale). (Figure 14-11.)

Retain breath for a moment. Fill with qi.

Bring your feet flat to the ground.

Repeat the entire sixth sequence two to three times.

Seventh Sequence

This series balances the:

- Gall bladder meridian
- Liver meridian
- Destructive influence: resentment, race, entitlement
- Positive influence: healthy boundaries, acceptance, faith

Breathe Naturally:

Focus on your eyes.

Look from deep within your head.

Focus and intensify your gaze (with no tension around the eyes or between the eyebrows, however).

Place your feet in a wide stance.

Keep your knees soft.

Your eyes should be intensely focused.

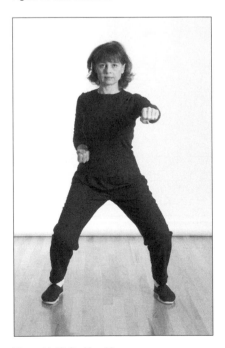

Figure 14-12: Position 12

Although the motion is important, the focus is in the eyes.

Make fists, palms up, below your shoulders.

Your elbows should be back behind your body.

Punch in slow motion:

Forward with one fist.

Rotating the fist as the arm extends.

Palm down when the arm is fully extended.

Reverse. (Figure 14-12.)

Repeat the entire seventh sequence two to three times on each side.

Eighth Sequence

This series balances the:

- Kidney meridian
- Bladder meridian
- Destructive influence: fear
- Positive influence: wisdom

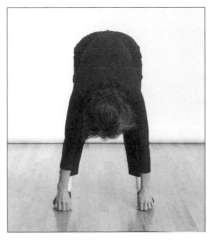

Figure 14-13: Position 13

This sequence is accomplished best with gentle sensitivity, as the inhalation and exhalation gracefully and gently guide the movement.

Stand with your feet a shoulders' width apart.

Exhale:

Slowly bend toward your toes.

Let your head lead the bend.

Let your spine roll down.

Take hold of a comfortable place on your legs or toes, if you can.

Pull *gently* for a further stretch. (Figure 14-13.)

Inhale-Exhale:

Breathe naturally and release to the stretch.

Your back is open. Take advantage of this by sending breath to your kidneys

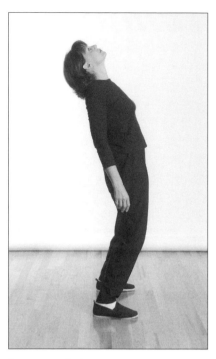

Figure 14-14: Position 14

Inhale:

After the last exhalation, inhale your-self up to standing.

The inhalation leads you to continue into a backward bend. Don't force it— be quite sensitive and gentle with yourself.

Inhale-Exhale:

The front of the body is open.

The lungs are open.

Fill them with qi. (Figure 14-14.)

On the last inhalation, come to standing.

Exhale, and repeat, continuing toward the toes.

Repeat the entire eighth sequence two to three times.

To further enhance the effect of the Eight Brocades, breathe and express the sound associated with the meridian pair:

Stomach and spleen: "Hooo"

Heart and small intestine: "Ho"

Bladder and kidney: "Chrroooeee"

Pericardium and triple warmer: "Suu"

Gall bladder and liver: "Shuuu"

Lung and large intestine: "Se-Ahh"

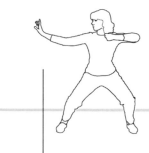

chapter 15
t'ai chi ch'uan
chi kung

MASTER TSUNG HWA JOU brought this form of qigong (he calls it, traditionally, chi kung) to the Western world through his excellent book *The Tao of T'ai Chi Ch'uan*. Earlier in his life he had suffered from an incurable illness, as mentioned in chapter 3. Devotedly learning and practicing t'ai chi ch'uan completely turned his health around. Going from frail to robust, he was determined to teach t'ai chi ch'uan to as many people as possible, in this way sharing the enormous gift he had experienced and hoping to assist others in the complex challenges of their lives. He did, indeed, fulfill that dream. After teaching in the West for decades, he finally put his vast amount of information into his book on t'ai chi ch'uan, intending it to be used as a textbook for any university or school wanting to add t'ai chi ch'uan to its curriculum. It is from this book I have taken the material in this chapter, presented here in a slightly adapted form.

Heng and Haah

Sound was incorporated into some forms of qigong. Two sounds used over time to incorporate qi were *heng* and *haah*. In the Chinese tradition of cloaked secrecy, they were kept secret until they were surreptitiously exposed in the lyrics of a song. Deciphering the lyrics opened up to the world the value of these words combined with breath and movement.

Master Tsung Hwa Jou presented them in a traditional qigong form, called here chi kung, which was developed to support the vitality required to master the martial arts. The sounds of heng and haah make this form unique, and it is useful to practice them before actually doing the sequences. Heng is said when the abdomen contracts. Master Jua suggests practicing three to five minutes at a time, three times a day, for a few weeks. Then take the next step.

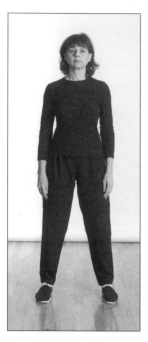

Figure 15-1: Position 1

The Sequence

Touch your dan tian.

Say "heng" and contract your abdomen.

Inhale.

Hold your breath, easily.

Say "haah," and exhale, relaxing your abdomen.

Repeat.

This is a breath-regulation technique that fills the body with a very refined and nourishing qi.

Position 1

Stand (or sit or lie if needed).

Place your feet shoulders' width apart.

Keep your knees straight and soft.

Hold your arms relaxed at your sides.

Relax into your body, head light as the imaginary string gently lifts it upward, extending and straightening your spine.

Breathe naturally and easily to the dan tian, and let your body prepare for the increase in breath and qi. (Figure 15-1.)

Position 2

Say "heng" while you float your arms up at your sides, and relax them as if they were supported by water, with the palms facing downward to Earth and the wrists relaxed and limp, which points the fingers down.

Float them up to shoulder height.

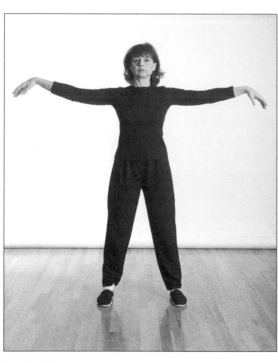

Figure 15-2: Position 2

Inhale through your nose, contracting your abdomen as you move your arms upward. (Figure 15-2.)

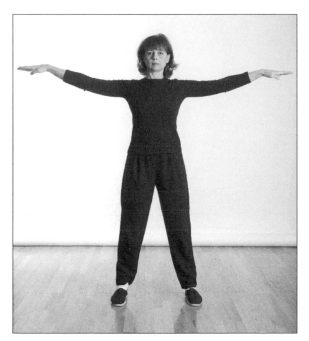 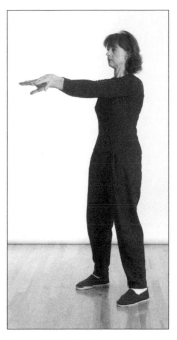

Figure 15-3: Position 3   Figure 15-4: Position 4

Position 3

Say "haah" while you exhale through your mouth, expanding your abdomen.

As you exhale, straighten your hands, initiating the movement at the wrists while the arms float submerged in the water.

Your wrists bring the fingers up.

Straighten your fingers, with your palms directed down toward Earth and your shoulders relaxed. (Figure 15-3.)

A good way to keep your shoulders relaxed is to feel the shoulder blade muscle pulling down as you extend your arms up and down.

Position 4

Say "heng" while you contract your abdomen.

Float your arms to extend to the front of your body.

Cross your right wrist over your left, palms facing down to Earth.

Your fingers are relaxed, though extended. Inhale, keeping your abdomen
   contracted. (Figure 15-4.)

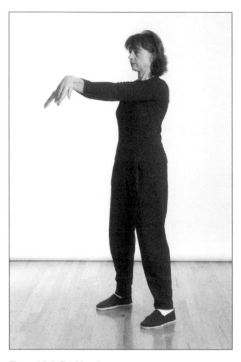

Figure 15-5: Position 5

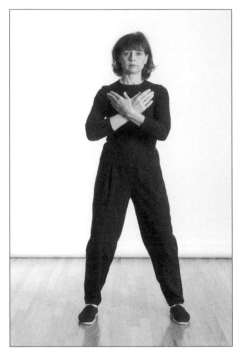

Figure 15-6: Position 6

Position 5

Say "haah" while you float your arms downward toward your body.

Your shoulders and wrists are relaxed. (Figure 15-5.)

Allow your palms to float down to face your body.

Exhale from your mouth.

Position 6

Say "heng" while you contract your lower abdomen.

Direct your hands in toward your body.

Your wrists remain crossed.

As you do the contraction and the wrist movement, simultaneously elevate
   your head, extending the spine. (Figure 15-6.)

Breathe naturally.

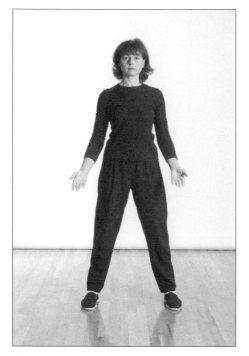

Figure 15-7. Position 7

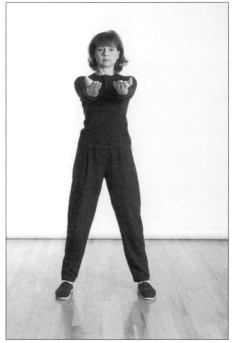

Figure 15-8: Position 8

Position 7

Unfold your arms and float them to the sides, palms forward.

Gradually straighten your knees simultaneously, inhale, and contract your abdomen. (Figure 15-7.)

Position 8

Say "haah" while you float your palms up toward heaven, and then out to the front of your body.

Bring your arms to the front of your body.

Exhale through your mouth. Your abdomen expands. (Figure 15-8.)

Position 9

Say "heng" while you contract your abdomen.

Inhale through your nose as you float your arms to your sides, at shoulder height.

Your palms are toward heaven.

Your fingers are relaxed, and your legs are straight, knees soft. (Figure 15-9.)

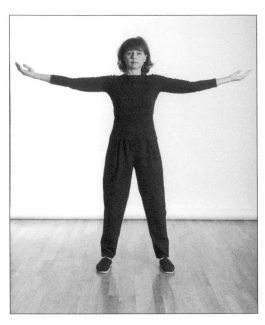

Figure 15-9: Position 9

Position 10

Say "haah" while you exhale through your mouth and expand your abdomen.

As you exhale, straighten your arms, open your hands, and extend your fingers.

Stretch your hands and fingers, palms up.

Relax on the water. (Figure 15-10.)

Position 11

Say "heng" while you contract your abdomen.

Lift your head upward, extending your spine.

Inhale through your nose with your abdomen still contracted.

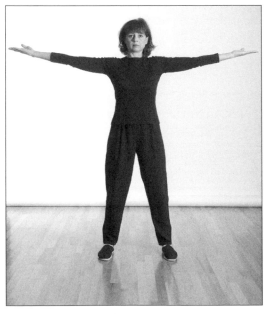

Figure 15-10: Position 10

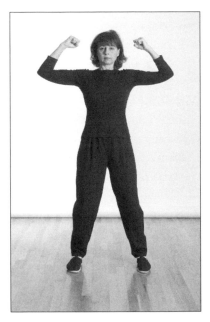

Figure 15-11: Position 11

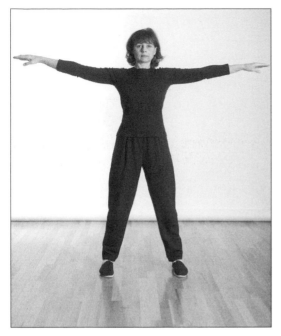

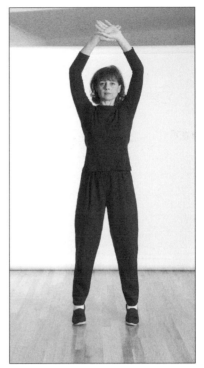

Figure 15-12: Position 12 (above)

Figure 15-13: Position 14 (right)

Make loose fists with your hands and bend your elbows, bringing the fists to face your ears.

Gradually turn your fists to face outward. (Figure 15-11.)

Position 12

Say "haah" while you exhale through your mouth and expand your abdomen.

Simultaneously straighten out your legs and float your arms to shoulder level.

Gently open your fists, relax your palms, and extend your fingers.

Your palms are downward. (Figure 15-12.)

Position 13

Say "heng" while you contract your abdomen.

As you inhale, abdomen contracted, bend your elbows, bring your fists to your ears, then extend your arms upward over your head, straight but not locked.

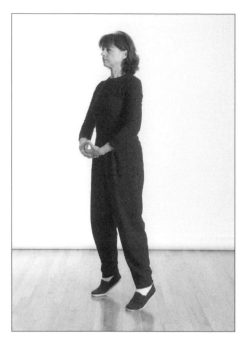

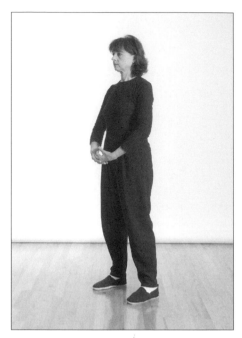

Figure 15-14: Position 15   Figure 15-15: Position 16

POSITION 14

Say "haah" while you open your fists, extend upward on your legs, and
stand up on your tiptoes (or, if sitting or lying down, point your toes and
think of standing on them).

Extend your arms and raise your hands over your head.

Cross your hands, right palm in back of left hand, with palms facing front,
and exhale through your mouth, abdomen expanded. (Figure 15-13.)

Position 15

Say "heng" while you remain on your toes and gradually lower your arms
in a circular fashion, so they naturally float together, with your hands
meeting at the dan tian.

The hands grasp each other, with the right palm under the back of the left
hand, thumbs touching.

As this movement occurs, inhale through your nose, expanding your
abdomen. (Figure 15-14.)

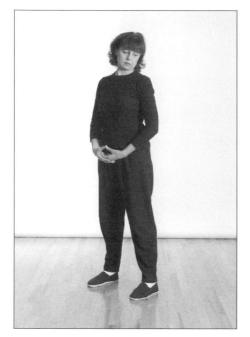

Figure 15-16: Position 17

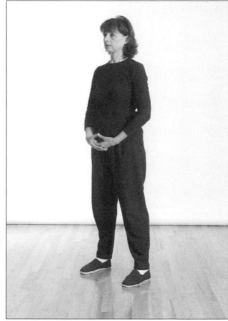

Figure 15-17: Position 18

Position 16

Say "haah" while you lower your body so your feet are flat on the ground, and exhale from your mouth, abdomen expanded.

Your hands stay laced at the dan tian.

Position 17

Say "heng" while you hold your entire body straight and still.

Lift your head upward, extending your spine. Moving only your head, turn and look over your left shoulder (with your hands still laced at the dan tian).

Inhale and contract your abdomen. (Figure 15-16.)

Position 18

Say "haah" while you exhale, expand your abdomen, and turn your head only as your body rests in steady stillness.

Look to the front, eyes soft and slightly unfocused. (Figure 15-17.)

Repeat the entire Position 18 sequence on alternate sides. Repeat three to five times. End on the right side.

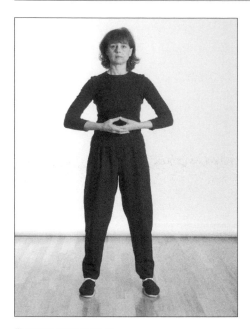

Figure 15-18: Position 19

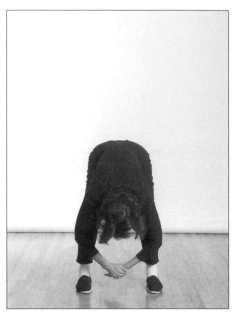

Figure 15-19: Position 20

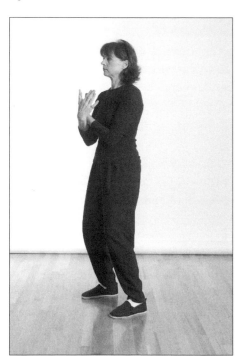

Figure 15-20: Position 21

Position 19

Saying "heng"

Contract your abdomen, and then inhale through your nose as you simultaneously lift your joined hands to your abdomen. (Figure 15-18.)

Position 20

Say "haah" while you exhale through your mouth.

Expand your abdomen.

Turn your palms face down and float them to the floor as you bend from the waist. (Figure 15-19.)

This entire Position 20 series should be repeated three to five times in sequence.

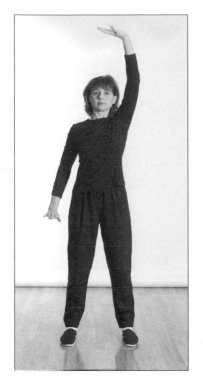

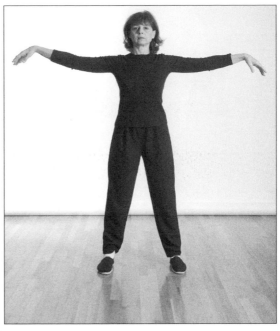

Figure 15-21: Position 22 (left)

Figure 15-22: Position 23 (above)

Position 21

Say "heng" while you contract your abdomen and inhale through your nose, while rising from the floor.

When erect, cross your wrists in front of your chest, right over left, with your palms facing your body. (Figure 15-20.)

Position 22

Say "haah" while you exhale through your mouth, expand your abdomen, lift your left palm flat to the sky, and press your right palm down, flat to the earth. (Figure 15-21.)

Repeat this entire Position 22 sequence three to five times by returning the crossed hands to your heart and extending your arms alternately. The first repeat sequence is the left wrist over the right, with right hand to heaven, left to earth. End with the right palm to the sky.

Position 23

Say "heng" while you contract your abdomen and inhale through your nose.

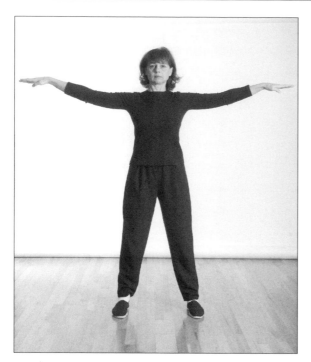

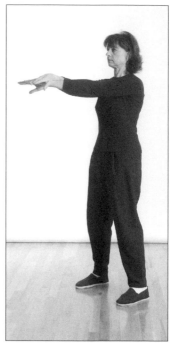

Figure 15-23: Position 24

Figure 15-24: Position 25

As you inhale, simultaneously lower your right arm and raise your left arm, until they are both evenly extended at your sides.

They are at shoulder height, palms down.

Your wrists are relaxed and limp. (Figure 15-22.)

Position 24

Say "haah" while you exhale through your mouth, expand your abdomen, and float your arms on water as you extend your hands and fingers with your palms facing toward earth. (Figure 15-23.)

Position 25

Say "heng" while you contract your abdomen as you inhale through your nose.

Float your arms toward the front of your body.

Place your right wrist over your left with your palms facing down toward earth. (Figure 15-24.)

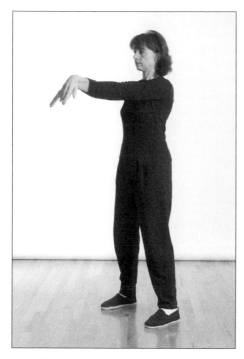

Figure 15-25: Position 26

Position 26

Say "haah" while you exhale through your mouth and expand your abdomen, allowing your wrists to relax, and float your hands downward, palms toward your body, fingers relaxed. (Figure 15-25.)

Position 27

Say "heng" while you contract your abdomen and inhale through your nose as you lower your hands, turning them toward your body.

When your arms have naturally floated down, they release in front of your thighs.

Position 28

Return your left palm to lie on your right palm, with your thumbs touching each other.

Straighten your legs and bring your joined hands up to your chest.

Position 29, Saying Haah:

Exhale through your mouth, expand your abdomen, turn your joined palms down to earth, let them separate, and float your arms gently to your sides.

Rest for a few minutes and let your body become accustomed to the new qi distribution.

part 5

deepening your practice

THE EXPERIENCE of deepening one's practice lies in the undisputable reality that the longer you do an Eastern discipline, the deeper and more meaningful it becomes. This may seem an odd state of affairs, since endless repetition is a negative experience. But in Eastern disciplines the repetition encompasses an intrinsic tool to enhance one's self-awareness and connection to omnipresence. This connection is one of rich endlessness. Practice facilitates the learning required to embody the movement. The movement lives within you. You settle in, and the deepening becomes a wide avenue of awareness available any time you practice.

The masters before us have demonstrated through poetry and mentoring that out of the deepening appears a loving humility and gratitude for all life.

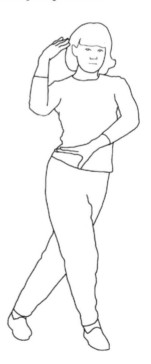

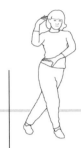

chapter 16

practice, finding your way to qigong

BEGINNER'S FRESHNESS is an ongoing goal of everyone who practices qigong—to be fresh in each day, like a child seeing it all for the first time, fully there, present. Practice will become for you an instrument for cultivating a beginner's attitude. The only requirement for gaining this clarity is commitment to practice.

You may be feeling a disadvantage at being a true beginner. On the contrary, you are in a great position. You know the possible value of qigong, so you are excited. Your curiosity motivated you to read this book and now to learn qigong. Excited, curious, and motivated are a triune for success. You are a true beginner, not knowing and ready. A teacher's dream come true.

As you pursue qigong, you will have three levels of development:

- Learning it
- Getting it down
- Perfecting it

Learning It

To begin the learning process, consider the word "practice." Practice as a verb means to train, to prepare. I am practicing qigong. Practice as a noun means training, but it also means a custom, a usage, or a vocation (such as the practice of medicine).

When you go to practice (verb) qigong, this use of the word immediately implies a need to do this in order to get somewhere else. To practice something conjures up a discipline of repetition taken on, sometimes reluctantly, to achieve a goal. But goal orientation is the antithesis of qigong. Qigong teaches a multilayered experience of presence. It's a bit like peeling an onion—with each layer peeled away, you get closer to the core. This demands no preparation or practice for any goal. Presence can't be a goal. You might as well try to get a handful of vapor. In qigong, having a goal would be just another excuse not to become present.

However, take the word "practice" and use it as a noun. This definition is a custom, a usage, a discipline, a vocation. I am doing my practice. The word creates, then, a whole new context. Practice as a noun means a creation or performance of something. This is the correct use of the word in regard to qigong. You take time for your qigong practice. You don't take time to practice your qigong.

A small, inconsequential point? I don't think so. We live in a very goal-oriented culture. Most of us have been raised in it, and these values permeate us as well as our culture. Qigong was born from the values of old China, values that placed much more emphasis on solving problems and setting goals after getting present and understanding the course and direction the qi was tak-

The practice will have an effect on your emotional life. Anger, depression, jealousy, and the like are very dense emotions, involving very coarse qi. In refining qi through qigong, even the most fledgling qigong practitioner begins to transmute the qi. Emotions will continue to be expressed, but only as necessary and appropriate to the situation. Self-acceptance and self-awareness gained through qigong reduce the inner friction, allowing a great deal of emotion to dissipate before it is expressed.

ing. It was understood that qi had the power to greatly influence health and life events. Therefore, only after understanding qi could one make any good goal-setting plans. First presence, then wisdom gained from presence. Without presence, how could one make wise decisions?

To be a student of qigong and to be open to all that it has for you, it is essential to develop the art of presence. Any tool you use to assist yourself in this effort is valuable. Words have a powerful effect on our conscious and unconscious mind. Use your word "practice" with wisdom. Release yourself from the verb "practice," which implies you're not there yet and you need to get somewhere else. Instead, do or exercise or enjoy or take time for or engage in or develop your qigong practice. As a learner you are finding the right times for

When practicing your dan tian breathing, let both your abdomen and your lower back relax and expand when you inhale. They will both settle back when you exhale. If this is a bit hard to get at first, put a hand on both your abdomen and your lower back, and move them with your breath.

qigong, and you are setting up the environment for your qigong practice. Both are important aspects for creating an ongoing desire for commitment and consistency in learning qigong.

Getting It Down

Your practice will become more integrated at this point. At first, when you're thinking, thinking, thinking about which foot goes where, the hand does this, or was it that . . . and now breathe in or out on this one—who has time to slide the mind on the breath? Every bit of mind is needed to serve the learning process! You benefit from this mental effort. You are using both sides of the brain together—right and left.

But then you become smoother in your qigong practice. The breath, the movement, even the mind settling in on the form, all start to integrate. There is a natural quality to the movement. You can *feel* when you are getting it right. Toward the end of this period of learning, you will also be getting a sense of who you are with qigong, how you like to do qigong, the form that is best for you, and the teacher and teaching style you enjoy. Qigong will be feeling like an ally, and doing practice will be as natural as sleeping and eating.

Perfecting It

The third stage, perfecting it, is lifelong. When the movements become you, the breath flows in those movements are like silk, without a thought; the movement and breath unite, and you and qigong are one. It is at this point that the

Qigong practice will give you a deeper understanding of the workings of things and where you fit in the harmony of all things.

mind work really takes off. There is no limit to what a trained mind can create. The freedom of knowing how to direct the mind is a unique outcome of the

*O*f your two biggest challenges in qigong, neither will be the actual movements. They will be: (1) finding time to do them and (2) benefiting enough that you will want more. The following is a very rough idea of a schedule you could use. Feel free to alter it to best suit you. If you start working with a teacher, the two of you will decide what is best.

Suggested Qigong Routine First Six Weeks

First Week

Morning: Standing (or sitting) meditation, 5 minutes

Evening: Relaxing visualization, 10 minutes

Second to Fourth Weeks

Morning: Standing meditation, 10 minutes

First eight steps of your chosen form, 10–15 minutes

(start with one step, and add a new step each day)

Evening: Relaxing visualization, 10 minutes

Breath work, 10 minutes (focus on the exhale rest point before you inhale)

Fourth to Sixth Weeks

Morning: Standing meditation, 10–15 minutes

The eight steps of your form

A new form or new steps, depending on the form you're working with.

Evening: Relaxation visualization, 10 minutes

Breath work, 20 minutes

Stress-releasing qigong stretches

third stage, a development that is not easily described. But it is a wonderful skill that enhances every conceivable area of life.

Moving from learning it to perfecting it requires a bit of self-knowledge. For all the folks who practice qigong in the West, there are probably just as many who have given up the practice, not because it wasn't good for them, but because taking the time for it became too problematic. Sometimes a well-thought-out plan is required to create the daily time your need for consistent practice. Sometimes, an understanding of what motivates you can help. Each one of us values things for different reasons. Combine qigong with something that has an intrinsic value for you, and it will become easier to create the time and actually do it daily.

If You Are Structured and Organized

Look carefully at your schedule. Examine your to-do list. Seek and find twenty minutes when qigong is workable. Carefully consider the addition. Is there another spot that might work better? When you have found the best spot, write qigong into your schedule.

If You Love Enticement and Rewards

When a problem occurs, say to yourself, "I am so glad I can do qigong after this. I will feel so much better after I have done qigong." After you have done your practice, you can have an aromatherapy bath. You can let yourself do qigong after you have finished your long day. Say: "Oh, tomorrow morning when I wake up, I can do qigong!" Basically, you can arrange and rearrange your thinking to put qigong practice in a reward position in your life.

You can create a very pleasant spot in which to do qigong. Enhance it with feng shui (see chapter 6), aromatherapy, light and color, or flowers. The only time you will be in this space is when you are preparing for qigong, doing it, or closing down from it. Qigong and the space become linked in your pleasure memory.

Read a book that you love, but only before or after qigong practice.

You Are a Nature Person

Find a place to do qigong that satisfies your need to be close to nature. Nature means a view, smells, and touch, and it can also mean just natural light. Your practice space can be in front of a window. Have a nature video play while you practice, set a time when you consistently open a window or door for fresh air, find a new way to enjoy your garden, enjoy a place in a park where you are safe and the surroundings are lovely. There are many ways to enhance your practice. Watch a bird, a cat, a dog, a leaf, and apply the movements you observe to practice. Nature has been the inspiration for qigong for thousands of years. It is a natural resource to turn to for a reason to make time to practice.

We are inspired by nature and love nature, but do we really nurture nature? Nature, Earth, needs nurturing, and this can be done in your practice. Simply form the intent to join nature in breath and movement, and even if you're just a beginner, you will feel nurtured and nurturing when you are finished.

You Revere Great Teachers and Being Able to Study with Them

Create a spot where you have something to remind you of the teachers who have brought qigong to you—a picture, a piece of old Chinese fabric, a flower, even just a votive candle in a safe container.

When you start your practice, relate to your area. Say thank you. Feel the humility of being able to learn from so many contributions from so many teachers. At the end of the session, turn again to this invisible entourage and give them thanks.

You can add a traditional element by starting or finishing with a cup of high-quality green tea, like Jasmine Downey Pearls.

Support your practice nutritionally. Eat very fresh food. Qi is in all living things, and food provides an important avenue for the absorption of qi. If you are hungry, having an organic apple, celery stalk, tomato, or fresh water before practice can provide more energy than a cookie, coffee, or a quick sandwich. Practice is better on a slightly hungry stomach.

You Like to See Your Progress

After one or two classes, take a video of yourself doing qigong. Then watch it or not, as you choose. Practice, knowing that you are trying to get better than the video. Six weeks later, take another video.

Put one hundred small pebbles or marbles in a jar. Take one out each time you practice.

You Are Social

Plan a class with a friend or a group of friends. Heck, get a whole group together and hire your own instructor. Then practice together.

You Love Silence and Don't Get Enough of It

Create silence to enfold your qigong. Turn off cell phones, and turn down or unplug your telephone. If there are traffic sounds, close the doors and windows. If there's no traffic, go outside. Wear earplugs if you need to, but give yourself silence while you do qigong. Start looking for places to practice that would also offer true silence. Qigong thrives as you acquiesce to silence.

You may miss practice every once in a while. You can make it up at a time different from your usual practice time. And if you are sick and unable to practice, visualize. With your eyes closed, sense yourself moving through your form. Sense the qi moving within you. This is actually a useful form of practice. It is a useful time to do Cuu si: healing visualization and techniques for concentration of the mind.

You Have Great Visualizing Skills

Allow your senses to become filled with a place that you love. When you have it in mind, step into your form and start to do qigong.

You Are Unsure about the Sequences

Get a qigong teaching video you really like. Dress for qigong, sit down with a cool drink, and watch the video. Imagine you are doing the movements right along with the tape. You might even become familiar enough with the tape that you can sense yourself doing the movements. This can often make you want to get up and do them. The sensing will make the form easier. Closing your eyes and seeing or sensing yourself doing it facilitates muscle memory and nerve stimulation.

You Have a Good Imagination

Imagine you are creating a screen made of energy, any color you like, around your qigong practice space. Circle the space with the screen, leaving the top open to heaven and the bottom to Earth. When you walk through this screen, it actually filters all the worry and concerns of the day out of the cells of your body. You step into your dedicated space feeling light, present, and free of daily cares. When you are finished, step out, and the cares will be with you again, but they may not be so worrying or consuming.

Your Life Is Filled with Responsibility, Maybe Even Burdens

The area before you enter your practice space is where you place your burdens. In qigong you will learn quite quickly where you carry the stress in your body. Say to yourself throughout the day: "I can put my burden down when I do qigong. I am looking forward to putting this down for a while, while I do practice." Before doing your practice, shake your shoulders, relax your hips, and let the tension out of your neck. Let it all go. Take a big breath, and as you exhale, let it fall to the floor in a big bundle. Step away from this bundle. It will wait until you get back. Do your practice and then step back to the bundle. Exhale, then inhale it back in. It won't be as heavy, and you will feel freer in the midst of your commitments.

You Are Spiritually Motivated

Let qigong be your time for meditation. Instead of the still, seated form you may be used to—yang inside and yin outside—let qigong now show you another side of meditation. Yin within, in peace, and yang without, the movement. Qigong can replace your twenty-minute sitting with a new approach.

The meaning of qigong will change for you as you deepen into the form. It will, after a time, become as essential to you as sleep and nutrition. Doing qigong will be a cornerstone of a day enjoyed and well lived.

 Qigong practices make the spine long and supple. The spine is the energy superhighway for qi. A supple spine means a vital body. Let your spine be like a rope, strong and flexible.

The traditional time for doing the practice is early morning, in the dewy grass. If you can do that, so much the better. Air is fresher in the morning. Your body is rested. The day awaits you, and qigong puts you right into correct alignment. Dew has traditionally been valued for its healing properties. Elder yogis walked in the dew to maintain their keen sight. Qigong first thing in the morning does feel great. It is universally regarded as the best time for practice to occur, but late morning, lunch break, afternoon, evening, or under the moon also offer unique benefits. It is a great idea to try out various times. The upside of this is that it will give you a good idea of what times you like best and why.

The downside is that it can keep you from establishing a predictable time. The human body thrives on variety, so the nervous system stays stimulated. But it also loves predictable structure. Qigong practiced at a certain time with consistent regularity provides both stimulation and structure. Find the time that works best for you. Make it a considered, well-thought-out decision. Commit to it. Make it work. Use a variety of techniques to make it appealing until it "takes." Then you are off and running into a future of better health, strong well-being, and a new sensitivity to qi.

Your Practice Schedule

What You Don't Need

Special equipment

Special clothes

Certain body type

Certain weight

Compatible philosophy

Understanding of qi

Sensing of qi

What You Do Need

A non-slip floor

Comfortable clothes

Non-slip shoes

Warming up

Love of feeling good

Willingness

Openness

Commitment

There is one sure way to success. Practice.

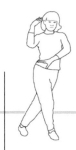

chapter 17

integrating qigong benefits

AS YOU DO QIGONG, unattended tense areas become obvious. If you have tight shoulders, stiff hips, or lower-back pain, it will surface. Each responds to the gentle nudging of qigong. Gentle flowing movements open joints and muscles to oxygen and qi. Over time, as the body relaxes, you will be at ease in yourself and with yourself. New pleasure in movement will suffuse all of your actions. This new freedom and pleasure infuses life with new vibrancy, more energy, brighter colors, fuller flavors. At this point it will be the most natural thing in the world to take aspects of qigong into your everyday life. But there is going to be some time between your initial practice session and the point at which qigong comes naturally to you, and during that time you will be learning how to integrate the benefits of qigong into your everyday life.

This chapter gives you ideas of good, bite-sized pieces of qigong that are easily applicable to life's challenges. These exercises will give you qigong as an assistant in your life, and the familiarity you gain with these techniques will greatly assist your practice.

Daily Integrations

First Warmup

There are two styles of qigong warmups. Both can easily transfer into your day. The first style consists of snippets of qigong that can be done both prior to doing qigong in the morning and in small installments interspersed through the day. Don't be self-conscious about getting up from your chair at work and doing a few lower-back de-stressors or a few focused spinal limbering rotations. Neck rolls done in an orderly sequence (not just a quick one thrown in between

Senior Moments?

The challenge of qigong may be learning the sequences. Any way that you include qigong snippets in your daily routine will enhance and improve your performance of qigong in the class environment. And remember, the nervous system loves the gentle stimulation of something new. Just the act of doing qigong is very beneficial. It really makes no difference how slowly or quickly you learn the complete form. The value is in the process.

the meeting and the car) drain mental tension and bring your body to the present. The heaven and earth stretch fits easily into a lunch break outside. For every minute one of these warmups takes, you will have at least an hour of benefit.

Second Warmup

The second type of qigong warmup is to do a sequential section of movements from a qigong form. Practice it in small, manageable bites. There are many opportunities for this, and more will occur to you as time goes by. Immediate benefit is derived from bringing qigong ease into your personal movements.

Elevating the Head

This exercise relieves sluggish thought, headaches, tight shoulders, tense jaws, third eyes.

An average head weighs about seven pounds. That is quite a bit of weight bearing down on the neck and shoulders. This weight alone can create neck

Are you pregnant? Qigong will provide a wonderful time of inner peace and tranquility. Since it balances qi, it is very useful for you and your baby.

and shoulder discomfort. But there is relief. Instead of feeling your weight bearing down, elevate your head. Pinch a few hairs at the top back of your scalp, where your part ends, and pull up gently. This will tip your head forward slightly. Allow your head to float and elevate. The spine will lift up and the shoulders relax down. As your head floats upward, let your breath slide down into the dan tian.

This positions the head correctly for qigong practice.

Soul for the Soles

This exercise is for lower-back tension, shoulder tension, tired legs, ungrounded feeling, shallow breath, feeling not present, racing mind.

Bring your awareness into the soles of your feet. Either in or out of your shoes, wiggle your toes. Move your foot. Imagine you are trying to lift up a carpet with your toes, curling them tightly against the ball of the foot. Relax your feet now, and imagine they are in contact with warm mud or sand. Imagine the gentle support and upward pressure you get from this surface. Stand, and now walk easily, not fast, with your awareness in your feet. (High-heels won't work, better go barefoot.) Imagine the support and traction. Breathe into the soles of your feet. Heighten your awareness. Continue to walk, maintaining the sense of solid, supportive contact with the ground. Now extend your awareness down the bubbling well. Root deeply into the earth. Keep on walking, and now bring your awareness to the soles of your feet and soul contact with the Earth. This pleasure walk can be done for one minute or an hour.

The value is in the grounding and releasing downward. This helps give you a feeling of secure footing during practice.

Easy Does It

This exercise is for lower-back problems, ungroundedness, tired eyes, trouble relaxing, shoulder tension, shallow breathing, emotional states, tension in the neck and shoulders.

Raise your head upward. Drop the bubbling wells into the earth as you place your feet about a shoulders' width apart. This is a turning action and can be used anytime you are looking around or reaching around for something—a mini-qigong break for you. Let your hips lead the movement. With your legs strong and stable, your feet grounded, you rotate your hips, and the upper body simply follows along. All the effort is in the hips, and the spine simply rotates as a result of the hips turning left and/or right. Your head elevates; your breath is easy and deep, and your torso is limp, just along for the ride. Stiffness born from unnecessary tension recedes. The stress in your head, neck, shoulders, and chest drains down and out.

This helps you develop the ropelike flexibility that prevents pain.

Walking and Aligning with Qi

This exercise is for stiffness, aching, tired legs and feet, tired brain, excessive emotions, feeling unattractive.

The spine is qi's superhighway. Many Eastern masters believe youth is dependent on a supple spine. A supple spine speeds qi through the body. A stiff spine slows the flow. Open the spine to supple movement by "growing a tail." Imagine you have a tail you are bringing along behind you as you walk. Make it any kind of tail you choose—a swishy tail, a heavy alligator tail, a peacock tail, a sleek leopard tail. Each image suggests its own set of feelings. Now take a walk, dragging your tail behind you. Keep your awareness in your spine and in the tail you are pulling along behind you. This opens the hips and grounds the legs for qigong.

Seed to Sun

This exercise is for shoulder stress, heavy head, stiff spine, achiness, ungroundedness, cold, tight or tired legs.

Bend your knees slightly, feet grounded, legs strong. Drop your chin to your chest, and let your head slowly pull down toward the floor. Bend at the waist and sort of curl down, limp, relaxed, stretching as you go. When you are bent over as far as is comfortable, arms dangling toward the floor, start your roll up. Imagine that you have a seed just planted in the base of your spine. As the seed sprouts, it goes straight up your spine toward the sun. You don't bring yourself up; the sprout does, until it bursts out of the top of your head. You can also do the roll back down while imagining that the sprout is withdrawing back to the base of your spine, and as it draws back into the seed, you release your upper body down, as your feet stay grounded, legs strong, knees soft.

This opens up flexibility in the torso, encourages the body-mind to strengthen its ability to create union through imagination, and grounds the legs and feet.

Eye Calming

This exercise is for eyestrain, headaches, neck tension, facial tension, tired eyes, shallow breath.

Our eyes anatomically extend to deep within the head, and yet our awareness tends to be on the surface of the eye. Deepening your awareness, to accept the fact that vision is born from deep in the head, allows the eyes to relax. Try this shift yourself. Move your awareness to the surface of the eye. It's like peering. Now shift your awareness down the optic nerve and let your vision emanate from deep within. That is seeing.

This helps the balance of the body, frees up the neck and head, and allows the energy centers in the body to function correctly.

Breath Integration

Because air is a constant component of life, breath integration exercises are easy, silent, unobtrusive, and very effective. The breaths we will be using are:

- Natural breath: The way you breathe without awareness
- Cleansing breath: Inhale through your nose, exhale through your mouth
- Tonic breath: Inhale through your mouth, exhale through your nose

There are more ways to guide the breath, but these are easy and quick to use in a busy life. (See chapter 10, "Breath Practice," for more discussion on breath and qi.)

Natural Breath

When you lie down on your back and breathe, this is natural breath. The breath flows into the pelvis/dan tian easily, and then the chest inflates. A fully inflated chest fills to about 80 percent of lung capacity. Forcing more air into the lungs simply increases body stress. To relieve inner tension, reduce worry, and get back into one's own timing rhythm, use the natural breath.

Feel your abdominal skin pressing against your clothing. Breathe into your abdomen and increase that surface pressure a bit. Notice as you breathe into the pelvis first, the chest rises from the bottom up, and the upper part of the chest lifts very little. It actually stays soft and responsive to the deeper rhythmic breathing. The exhaled breath just pours out effortlessly. Once again the inhalation flows deep into the pelvis/dan tian, lifts the chest from the bottom up, and then rolls out.

Feeling too emotional? Let the sound of the emotions come out when you exhale, then fill yourself with fresh qi and air. Eventually the new qi will replace the coarser qi in which the emotions are residing. You will feel more resolved and emotionally clear. This makes deep, easy breath familiar, so blending the qigong breath with your natural breath.

Cleansing Breath

This exercise is for when you are feeling too emotional, when your mind is cluttered, when you experience knots of tension, bad feelings, uncomfortable thoughts, depression.

Everything is made up of qi. That is true for your flesh, bones, blood, thoughts, and emotions. Qi is like a flow of water that goes where it is directed. Unpleasant emotions and thoughts—anger, jealousy, envy, and greed—flow in coarse qi. Love, peace, equanimity, and other such feelings flow in more refined qi. Everyone has the potential to include both types of qi and have access to a range of feelings. To refine feelings, thoughts, and emotions or to just plain get rid of them, the cleansing breath is great. Focus on what you want to lift up to a higher thought form or dispense with completely. For instance, lift anger up to become boundary setting, transform envy to self-satisfaction, greed to satisfaction. Or just breathe out the anger, envy, or greed. Focus on or fill yourself (you may already be filled to overflowing with the feeling) with the feeling or emotion. Inhale and fill up more. Open your mouth, open your throat, and demand that the emotion flow out on your exhaled breath. Again inhale through the dan tian up to the chest. Feel the emotion rise within. Exhale as forcefully as you choose. You can couple the exhalation with an appropriate sound as well. Dump that coarse qi, loaded with unwanted emotion, out of your body. Fill up with fresh qi and repeat until you are once again balanced and clear. A great tool for anyone.

This exercise strengthens the connection between the body and qi's tremendous potential for balance.

Tonic Breath

This exercise is for when your energy level is low, when you experience depression, difficulty focusing or getting ready for exertion, heavy-heartedness, or when you just feel as if you're coming down with something.

This breath will energize you with oxygen and qi. Be sure not to breathe too fast or too shallowly. Use slow, steady breathing. This is good after the cleansing breath. Dispel the unwanted with the cleansing breath, and then tone with the tonic. Dispel what you don't want, and tone with what you do want. Focus on what you want to draw in—patience, kindness, endurance, and the like—and do a few more tonic breaths than cleansing. The tonic breath on its own tones the nervous system, energizes the muscles, and prepares the body for a next step. The next step is decided by you—a walk, a run, a difficult conversation, or, if you are exhausted, it can give you enough energy to finally go to sleep.

Do three to twelve breaths.

For the breath exercises to achieve maximum benefit, find the best clean air available. Outside is best, but not essential, particularly if you live in an air-polluted environment. Try to be near negative ions, which are beneficial to the body. These are provided when air circulates over a body of water, and negative ion machines are also available. Wear clothes that allow the breath to flow unrestricted by a tight waistband. The breath exercises can also be greatly enhanced by any view. If a view is not available, then use your mind again and think of the horizon, and the blue skies, stretching far away. This helps ramp up the quantity and quality of qi you are internalizing.

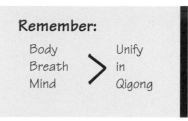

Remember:

Body   Unify
Breath   >   in
Mind   Qigong

These breaths are easy to do in an unobtrusive way. You will draw no unwanted attention to yourself as you do them. Taking a mini-break to utilize them accomplishes several important things. You learn to remind yourself to center in yourself and regain yourself as outer stress increases. You gain personal, practical information about their value for you. You reinforce your familiarity with qigong for daily use. You improve your breath skill for your practice. The best things in life are free, and the best of these is air, with oxygen and qi. You will become more and more attuned to walking, not in emptiness, but surrounded by a life-giving environment.

Three Basics

Your body provides the only tool you need to work with the three basics. Since these three reminders are subtle, you can embody them boldly and dance or subtly walk through a crowd. Qigong fits into enhancing life as smoothly as a smile.

- Relax into the form (your body's bony structure).
- Float through the movement.
- Keep your joints open.

These can become as much a part of your life as you choose. The tremendous value of remembering "Relax – Float – Joints Open" is that it relieves stress that has built up in your body. But even more important, it teaches you how to prevent stress from eroding your inner tranquility.

For instance: Traffic has come to a halt, and you are a bundle of frustration. Don't turn up the music or turn on the news. Take a deep dan tian breath, shift your weight, become more comfortable, and relax. Let the breath float in and out; let the joints open. Be in the experience. Choose to benefit from it and from qigong. Now turn up the music or turn on the news.

Running the Meridians with Your Mind

This exercise will help you:
- Maintain general good health
- Relieve minor pain
- Be qi aware throughout the day
- Experience the way that qi follows thought

This exercise is more advanced and offers tremendous advantages. It will increase the flow and improve the balance of your qi highways. You will be taking a meaningful step toward guiding qi with your mind. You will be practicing the form of qigong that combines movement, sound, and mind guidance to promote good qi flows in the body.

Get a map of the course of the meridians throughout the body. The Touch for Health Foundation in Pasadena, California, has a great book covering just this subject.

Start with the stomach meridian. Trace over your skin with your fingers the path of the meridian from face to toe. Now while your skin is still reverberating from your fingers' touch, pretend or imagine that you can see the meridian. The flow starts at the head under the eye and stops on the toe. Now move on to your spleen, and so on, until you have completed the circle of meridians and are back at the stomach. This takes a while, but has a powerful effect. Once you have the sequence, you can run them as needed during the day—and perhaps even more important, you will understand the reason for the movements in the form of qigong that addresses these flows directly.

Rocking and Rolling

This exercise improves balance, helps you regain centeredness and give up control, redefines grounding, and improves emotions.

Stand with your feet a shoulders' width apart for a stable base, with your toes forward if possible. With very small movements, roll forward onto the balls of your feet and back onto your heels. You will sense a midpoint where you feel well balanced. Not too far forward or too far back on the heels. Your knees should be easily soft. Now, just as imperceptibly, shift your weight from the right side of your feet to the left side, until once again you find a point of balance. These two balance points will merge, and you will be perfectly balanced.

Drop the qi from the bubbling wells downward as you adjust to this feeling of being balanced and ready.

This is the perfect qigong starting position.

Clearing-Your-Head

Walk

This exercise is for mental confusion, overwork, feeling overwhelmed or stifled, trying to make a decision, balancing meridians.

Stand balanced, weight on the right leg (yang) and no weight in the left leg (yin). Keeping the weight on your right leg, lift your "empty" left leg up and out into a step. Now the left leg gets heavy (yang), as you shift your weight to the left leg. The right leg becomes empty, and you bring it forward and take a full step. Now the right leg fills and takes the weight, and the left empties to take the step. And so on. This may be slow walking at first, but it is well worth becoming familiar with the movement. Once you get it moving, let your arms swing lightly at your sides.

This will create a much better understanding of guiding qi in your body during practice.

Do you have children? Don't bother teaching them the form. If they have a natural interest, they will copy you and follow along as best they can. This is actually the purest way to learn qigong. Many Chinese qigong practitioners learned it this way. It is fun to remind a child to exhale anger and make sounds, too.

For children who are highly sensitive to the energy levels of their surroundings, qigong can provide a good format for talking about qi, qi fields, and how the child perceives energetically. This can be a big help to an energetically sensitive child, who can then work with the concept of boundaries to protect his or her precious sensitivity.

At Ease

This exercise is for when you're under pressure, when you need to recenter, need to slow down, or need a break.

Relax as best you can. Inhale, drop your jaw, and let your mouth open slightly. Let the exhalation just flow out. Inhale into your pelvis and exhale again. Do this until you have carved a space for yourself, then reengage with the outside world.

This polishes your skill at inhaling deeply and then releasing into the movement.

Bull's-Eye

This exercise is for any area that is uncomfortable.

Focus on the area. Use your mind to create the sense of breathing directly into and out of that area. Keep the breath working at releasing the discomfort in the area until there is some relief.

This has a very positive effect on the skill of focusing the mind and breath.

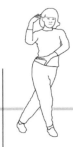

chapter 18

expanding your
knowledge of qi

Q I IS TO LIFE what numbers are to mathematics. One creates the other. Without numbers, mathematics would simply cease to exist. Without qi, life simply ceases to exist.

A person can explore the less complex elements of math (2 + 2 = 4, for example), and be satisfied, just as a person can simply breathe each day and feel fine. Another person will pursue a curiosity about numbers, eventually achieving a great understanding—numbers are the communication of the universe. Numbers and qi are the universal language and energy of life, respectively.

What qi knowledge provides is an excellent tool for taking charge of our emotions. Balanced emotions support a tranquil mind. A tranquil mind is a wise guide through life's challenges. A tranquil mind is filled with knowledge about qi and how to guide it to improve oneself and increase one's quality of life.

Unlocking the secrets of qi, as with mathematics, requires only curiosity and exploration. You can simply breathe and let it be

Times When Qi Is Refined

☞ A close talk with a friend

☞ A glass of water at the perfect time

☞ A good meditation or prayer time

☞ A glance at a lovely sight

☞ A good, deep breath

☞ A decision made, and followed through on, to find the joy in each event, to become satisfied, to seek the highest level

☞ A commitment to know another person well

☞ Your list: _____

_____

Seven Types of Qi

Breath qi, from air

Food qi, from nutrition

Birth qi, which we are born with

Inner qi, within the body

External qi, extending from the body

Nutritive qi, in meridian flows

Protective qi, which guards against external problems

enough or strike out and explore this universal force with a curiosity fueled by a love for the exquisite subtleties within flourishing, blooming life. Unlike mathematics, which is explored through books, formulas, and mental exchange, the theory of qi can only be explored through experience. The exploration of books, ancient manuscripts, and the teachings of modern-day masters is powerful and inspiring. That the ancient art was valuable for thousands of people is evident. But to know qi personally, you must have an experience, a personal experience, of sensing it.

Part of this sensing is the intimate awareness that your health and well-being are improving, your emotions are balancing, and your sense of steady groundedness is increasing. Another part of expanding your sense of qi is being able to discern the types or frequencies of qi available. This is a subjective process, and an extremely valuable one.

Never aloof, qi permeates all of life. We make the choice about our level of involvement. In making the choice to know more, we decide how to engage and encourage qi. What are the best qi sources? Can qi assimilate in a variety of ways?

There are two sources of acquired personal qi: breath and food. There are three sources of interactive qi: nature, human interaction, and spirit.

This assimilation is something we have experienced many times without realizing the contribution qi makes to these moments. When we unexpectedly come upon a commanding view of nature, we experience the silence of awe, the moment of pure connection to the view, the astonishing sense of renewal—all of our senses are involved in the perception of the view. But that moment of oneness and connection is the contribution of qi. Qi is the connecting medium. Qi is the fabric that draws us into oneness.

A fabulous meal of wonderful food exquisitely prepared, delightfully presented, and eaten with relaxed enjoyment produces a pause at the end. This satisfaction, tranquility, and complete well-being are the result of qi's effect. Food fills up your senses. Qi brings the tranquil well-being that takes that satisfaction and transforms it into a spiritual experience. Qi expands the senses. The life force contained in the food, now internalized in the body's energy flows, spreads pleasure, nurturing, and tranquility throughout the body. The presence of high-quality qi provides these delights. The best things in life are free, and they are because of qi.

When you look at a beautiful view, your senses perceive it, but what gives you the experience of connection to it? Qi flows through it and you. Qi is giving you the connection.

Human companionship is another arena for the cultivation of qi. Great company, laughter, and good conversation create the emotional qi environment that elevates everyone involved. The connections between members of the dinner party become increasingly warm and accepting. Humor and pleasure flow everywhere. Add to this mix great music and lovely fresh flowers, and these moments of satisfaction last for a lifetime as treasured memories to be tapped into and restored at will. Good energy.

Conversely, an unfortunate combination of people, who mix like oil and water, has reduced many an evening to a miserable missed opportunity. Again, qi is the reason misconnection occurs. Without qi, each person would be alone in his or her experience—no successful sharing. The reason a difficult dinner guest can ruin a great event is that human qi creates a powerful energetic exchange. A good combination creates the frequency of heaven. A destructive combination, hell.

Unless human qi is understood and guided, human interaction leaves many outcomes to chance. A skillful diplomat can upgrade the emotional climate. This promotes a frequency of qi that supports camaraderie. This is an acquired skill and available to anyone curious enough to explore the deeper arenas of qi.

Nature, nutrition, and human interaction are three fertile areas ripe with the potential for expanding qi awareness.

Nature and Qi

Being nurtured by nature's inspiration is an easy way to rebalance and restore qi. Qigong practice in these environments is a particularly powerful tonic. But it can be taken one step further. Enhance the experience further by nurturing nature back. Appreciate the extraordinary ways nature surrounds and cares for us. Then increase this qi frequency and flow. Use qigong as a dance to nurture nature. Nurture from your heart what you sense around you.

Receive inspiration, experience awe, grow gardens for beauty, but don't forget to nurture in return. It benefits nature as profoundly as it elevates qi. This frequency of qi strengthens the heart and bestows a deep sense of personal relationship to the beauty of life.

Nutrition and Qi

Live food carries qi; dead food has greatly reduced qi and carries the emotional residue of its life. This does not mean we should eat only raw foods. What this means is that the quality of the food is critical, plant or animal. Was it nurtured, fed live nutrients, and harvested, or slaughtered, with care? Or were the plants raised in soil that had diminished nutrients and yanked out of the silent ground by a noisy, violent machine?

Was the animal happy in its existence? Its state of life affects the qi frequency in its body, dead or alive. Animals that are miserable and die afraid leave a residue of these qi frequencies in their bodies. People who eat these animals are affected subtly but powerfully by these residual qi frequencies. An animal treated well and killed humanely will carry no low-frequency qi. Free of misery, fear, and the hopelessness of neglect, it is filled instead with the high-quality qi of nature's most contented creatures. Eating the meat of these animals elevates qi frequency at the critical body-building, cellular level. Choose animals, fish, and fowl whose meat harbors the contentment that they felt throughout their lives.

We are what we eat, and we are the frequency of the qi we eat in live food or the qi residue left in dead food. With this well in mind, visit grocery stores with a new, discerning eye. Fresh, colorful, flavorful foods are filled with qi. Preparing them in a timely fashion brings them to your table filled with life.

Preparing food with care and nurturing it into the perfect state to be eaten need not be time-consuming. The value is not in having a picture-perfect meal straight out of a magazine. The value is in the level of nurturing you are putting into the grilled cheese sandwich. Is the bread fresh, are the grains healthy, and is the cheese from happy and healthy cows? The grilled cheese sandwich that satisfies these requirements will carry a higher qi content than a full dinner of factory-farm beef, old vegetables, and desserts full of processed sugar. This approach to nutrition requires not a moment of extra work. It only needs awareness when picking out foods, and perhaps a change of markets.

There is no need to become austere. The body gravitates toward its own healing. Given good qi-filled food, it will begin to crave these foods. The desire for the previous diet will wane. A good rule of thumb for kids who are attracted to poor-quality food by the lure of advertising is: 80 percent good for your body, 20 percent fun for your tongue to taste.

Human Connection

This is maybe the easiest area in which to sense qi frequencies. We all have had times when we felt something from another person—anger, impatience, warmth, worry—that was not picked up through body clues, but through the "ethers." This is qi sensitivity, an ability to sense the qi field around the person and the dominant emotion emanating from that field. For this reason it is wise to choose your friends with care. Human qi interaction is so dynamic that we cannot escape its intertwining, but we can choose to be with people who don't "bring us down," diminishing our frequency. We can prefer to be with people who "brighten our spirit" to an upgraded frequency.

The qi fields between two people begin to interact and exchange energy the moment they meet. There is no way to stop this. It is a fundamental piece of human interaction. But through qigong practice, it becomes easier to discriminate within the qi exchange and consciously create qi boundaries to prevent an undesirable energy exchange from occurring—or you may wish to open completely the channels of qi exchange that allow a sought-for frequency to come through.

*C*hinese masters learn qigong to unify three principles:

Sexual Energy – Jing

Qi

Spiritual Energy – Shen

China has traditionally revered men with the balance that ensures a wise, strong, and active person, with the sexuality/ life/spirit inherent in all people.

This interaction reaches its peak of movement in sexual encounters. From the first moment of attraction, the qi fields become more alive. Excitation increases in both people. As the exchange progresses, the qi can reach extremely high frequencies, and in sexual exchange when love has guided the encounter, the individuals' spirits create a sexual-qi-spiritual experience.

Using Qi to Shape Your Interactions with Others

Very often we are confronted with a person who is unpleasant. Aggression, whether passive or active, is coarse qi, dense and undesirable. Unless you're in danger, it is seldom practical to spin on your heel and walk away. Instead, a coping mechanism is needed to deflect the coarse qi, engage as needed, and then retreat when possible.

All of these exercises are examples of commanding qi with your mind. The soul of cooperation, qi responds to your will. Practice these exercises in private so they are at your fingertips when you need them. Imagination is the tool of the mind in these exercises. Imagination in these cases makes the experience real, because you aren't creating fiction, you are guiding qi.

Imagine or sense that you have a mirror surrounding you, about an arm's length away. However, the mirror is not reflecting you. You have it turned out, and it is reflecting life around you. Demand that the mirror reflect back to the sender all qi that is not in your best interest. In addition, order the mirror to provide qi screening so that you can receive that which is in your best interest. This mentally guided qi field allows you to keep the qi area next to your body—sometimes called the aura—compatible and nourishing for you.

When another's coarse qi permeates this qi field close to you, it can create emotional havoc. This makes it impossible to respond according to your true nature, and instead you have a defensive response. Your qi field has been attacked, so a defensive response is understandable, but it seldom improves the situation. Better to be proactive. Protect your emotional qi field first and foremost. The mirror will do its job as you have demanded. Take a breath. Ground yourself through the bubbling wells, and choose a response that pleases you. It is a wonderful empowerment to realize you can protect yourself emotionally without raising a finger.

How can you help another to repair a qi wound that you have generated with an unkind word or aggression? This requires several steps. First is a recognition and acceptance of your role. To avoid shame, accept your behavior. You are not perfect. You are, like all others, learning. To be imperfect does not mean accepting shame. You are learning, and you are fine. Apologize to the other person for your actions. The next step is a timing issue. When the other person demonstrates openness to you, simply send love. Qi warmth sent to others, often in silence, will heal the wound in their field.

How can you support another? Take a deep breath and fill your qi field. Take a few more breaths and fill the qi field to overflowing. Demand that your qi field expand to embrace the person. This qi movement can be done by imagining your field creating two arms that go around the person's legs and feet, in a gentle qi-embrace. If you love this person, fill the qi arms with love by simply sending love into them. It's so easy, it's amazing we haven't been doing this since childhood. The length of time you engage in the qi hug is up to you. If you feel any sense of discomfort, pull the arms back and let any qi the hugging arms picked up be filtered out at the edge of your qi field. The edge of the qi field that surrounds you is like an energetic membrane that can easily tighten and protect the inner environment from unwanted, coarse qi.

To Touch Another Long-Distance

Reaching out and touching someone can happen easily using your qi field. Think of the person (you can do this with pets, plants, trees, etc.). Get him or her clearly in mind. Feel what you want to impart, and now just send it to the person, holding him/her in mind. The qi field of connection knows no time or space, and it is more complex and accurate than the phone lines. Your message will connect with the person you've chosen.

A word of caution: If you are sending something the other does not want—for example, ill wishes, self-centered desires, longings of unrequited love—the qi will be rejected, and sent back magnified sevenfold. If you send something out and you feel worse, this may be what has happened. So resend it, but change the address. Send it to anyone who can benefit from it. There is certainly someone who needs a bit more anger to change a terrible situation, who needs to be more self-centered to stop a cycle of doormat behavior, or someone whose heart will soften when feeling the unrequited love. Qi connects us all as one. We just need to learn how to use this field intelligently and skillfully.

Using the Membrane for Inner Security

A crowded environment can be tedious, or downright threatening. There is a simple qi trick that helps generate internal privacy and security. Demand that the outer edge of the qi field cozy right up to your skin, everywhere. Draw the membrane close, especially over areas that hurt (shoulders, neck, lower back) or feel uneasy (chest, thighs, forehead). If needed, densen the membrane, making it thick, like leather. Then when you are on your own, exhale as you expand the qi field. Shake your shoulders, take a deep breath, and feel the space that now exists between your body and the membrane. This is a very important space and completely under your control. Do what feels good to you. Fill it with colors, make it fluffy or smooth—you call it. It is your own, private qi space.

Your Personal Space

Qi courses through your body. It fills the world and universe, and it does something else of great importance. It provides you with your own space, your own, private space given to you by the universe. This is a space where you have complete control, not of life, but of your own quality, the quality of person you are in life.

Many people make a genuine effort to be an evolving, improving person. If the effort is made without understanding the alliance that qi provides, the successes are often diminished. The qi field that surrounds you is your buffer from life. It is the qi frequencies that nurture you. It is you, in the qi sense. To take charge of this intimate field is life-enhancing.

You shower, comb your hair, and brush your teeth each morning. Now add clearing your qi field. The easiest way to do this is to demand it to clear in the shower. It is particularly important to let the water run over the crown of your head, even if you wear a shower cap. Then at the finish of the shower, imagine all the colors that appeal to you on that day filling the entire space between your body and the outer qi membrane. The membrane is usually about an arm's length away, all around your body, a bit like an egg in shape. You are the yolk, and the qi field, the white.

We are each born with a certain level of qi available to us. What we are born with is what we have our entire life. Some are born with an amazing constitution, others with fragile health that requires vigilance. Whatever your inborn qi level, qigong will benefit you. High-energy people will learn to relax, an important aspect of any life, and low-energy people can gain a magnificent tool for strengthening their constitution.

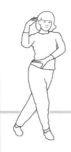

chapter 19

teaching qigong to others

Q IGONG MOVEMENT has two basic modes of expression: systematized qigong (the subject of this book) and instinctive qigong.

Systematized Qigong

The requirement for learning a system is that it be taught by a qualified person trained in the system. For a system as old and evolved as qigong, it takes devotion to training and personal growth to make one a qualified practitioner. The art of the teacher comes after this training and growth.

This is not to say that qigong has only been taught by trained and qualified practitioners. Anyone who wants to can claim to be a qigong teacher. In China, where transmission of qigong has been strictly controlled, the art has not merely maintained its original level of quality, but surpassed it. It has a history of evolving and then transcending itself, due to its steady commitment to excellence and quality.

In the Western world, there is no such cultural commitment to qigong. Without meaning to, enthusiastic but inadequately trained teachers have reduced the value to be gained from qigong. It is hard to take another where one has not been. Inadequately trained teachers just haven't been acquainted with qi and qigong long enough to be qualified practitioners. And they usually do not have an Asian master teacher who is the end product of a lineage of master teachers.

Trained teachers are certainly available, but you must make a commitment to go where they are. To do justice to the form and what it is capable of imparting, these trips are essential.

Instinctive Qigong

There is another basic qigong, however. This qigong has not been systematized. It has no masters who teach the essential, intricate steps. It is as valuable as the other basic qigong, but quite different. This is instinctive qigong. Instinctive qigong can be shared and enjoyed with anyone. You can lead the beginner as a guide. It is a marvelous way to share qigong. It ripens the health of the body with greater qi awareness. No intricate system of learning is being compromised. Best of all, you get to satisfy your very sincere desire to share your enthusiasm and newfound skills. Often this occurs in the second stage, when all the prerequisites for being a good teacher are present except a long history of practice and a mentor relationship with a master.

Instinctive qigong is not a form that follows any known type of movement. It is not emotional release movement. It is not required to be graceful, composed, or agile. When teaching instinctive qigong, give the first few minutes to explaining this.

There are four general stages for the qigong practitioner:

☞ First Stage: Just learning. "This is fabulous. I want to tell everyone." Still learning.

☞ Second Stage: Enough skill to practice autonomously. "This is fabulous, and I am fabulous. I want to teach this to everyone." Almost there.

☞ Third Stage: True deepening into the form. "I don't really know that much after all." Still learning.

☞ Fourth Stage: Union with qi. "I am here, engaged, and it is enough." Presence.

The First Freedom

Withdraw from the structure and demands of the outer world. Release any obligation of effort. The entire focus will be within. Closing the eyes in preparation for this is a useful tool for leaving the outer world for a while.

The Second Freedom (five minutes)

Standing. Now you can teach a system, the only one in this type of qigong.

Begin in Qigong Stance:

Feet together, or if balance is a problem, a shoulders' width apart, or one in front of the other. The goal, basic to qigong, is to ground to the earth. Feel the

Because repetition is the most negative state in the universe, instinctive qigong provides a wonderful retreat from qigong practice that has reached a point just prior to breakthrough. When it seems as if you are doing nothing but repeating and getting nowhere (which is actually not true—you are progressing invisibly), instinctive qigong can be exactly the right thing to help you open up for the next level.

feet connect to the earth. Explain about the bubbling wells. People can massage them prior to the stance. Lead step by step:

Relax.

Settle down.

Keep the knees soft.

Sink down in the pelvis.

Elevate the head.

Hold the back relaxed and easily straight.

Breathe to the dan tian.

Relax the arms.

Elbows should be soft and rounded.

Hold the palms facing each other.

Let each person find his or her place of balance.

Eyes may be either open or closed.

The stance is without effort.

The breath is easy and rolling in and out of the dan tian.

The mind is in the breath, feeling the abdomen expand and relax.

Instinctive qigong is the perfect expression of utter simplicity and trust.

The Third Freedom

Settle upon a time to end the session, and then briefly explain that you are keeping track of the time. You will let everyone know when it's time to stop. They are free to move in time and space with no concern for linear time. This helps free busy, preoccupied minds. As long as the mind knows it can reengage with the outside world at a specific time, it will go on "vacation" for awhile.

Many exercises and work-outs emphasize the strengthening of the outer muscles first, strengthening the heart and opening breath. All of these are great, but they overlook the importance of strengthening the core of the body first—the muscles of the circle of the foot and the inner legs, deep in the pelvis, along the spine, and at the back of the neck. It is these muscles that form the inner core of strength or weakness. Injury is far less likely to happen if this core is strong and qi-filled. Instinctive qigong engages this core. The whole body is the beneficiary.

The Fourth Freedom (five minutes)

Embracing effortlessness allows the inner movement of qi to flow into the bones, nerves, and muscles, generating its own movement as it shifts to the external world, becoming visible in movements of the body. This is a completely unself-conscious expression of personal movement and best done in an environment of privacy and acceptance.

The inner flow of qi externalizing creates unique movement—oddly slow, rhythmic, and bobbing are some of the movements that can be experienced. The arms will flow with the movement coming from the core of the body and moving out. The feet may stay grounded in one place, or the legs and feet may lift and move. The spine, like a limber rope, responds to the unique internal qi-feeling movement. The head, easily elevated, bobs, rolls, or stays unmoving. All are expressions of being moved by qi. The mind is in a state of suspension, vacationing.

The Fifth Freedom (five to ten minutes)

Encourage each person to feel qi and express movement only for herself/himself. In this state of awareness, the spirit is expanding out through the body to beyond. The core is strong, the root of the spirit, grounding spirit in the body. The spirit expands to the horizon all around. To the blue skies all around. To the cosmos and beyond. Spirit expands from the core.

After a few minutes, draw the spirit back, through the forehead, through the head. Your spirit returns to the body. Feel the skin, the natural boundary. Feel the feet deep in the earth, like a sequoia's roots. Feel the tranquility brought back by the spirit. Feel the sense of spaciousness. The mind is suspended in a state of emptiness and fullness. . . .

The Sixth Freedom (three to ten minutes)

Settle into this state of quiet. Your body will feel different. There may be subtle movements, vibrations, or a sense of openness or restriction in certain areas. Allow these sensations to simply be in your awareness. Your breath continues to roll in and out of the dan tian. Each sensation is a dynamic area. Each sensation is a place where the qi wants to flow toward the external world and is not freed up. Continue to settle and sink into the myriad of sensations.

The Seventh Freedom (ten minutes)

There will come a point when these inner sensations can externalize. With very little external expression, multiply the sensation within. For instance, you feel tension under a shoulder. Exaggerate it, magnify it. Does your arm want to swing? Does your head want to roll? Does your back want to move? What movement wants to occur as you exaggerate the tension? Follow the movement mentally. This is the qi seeking and finding gateways to the external world. As the qi moves, the shoulder will release tension on its own.

One movement will lead to another. Let your body express itself.

You may feel emotional awareness and mental perceptions flow through you as you express the movement outwardly. They are a part of the instinctive qigong experience. This is the qi moving. All the movements of qi are freeing—mentally, emotionally, physically, and spiritually. Stay on your feet and feel the ground. Don't leave your body, but expand from your body. The core is filled with qi extending through bones, nerves, and muscles into the external world. The mind remains suspended.

Things to be aware of:

- The feet stay grounded, stepping very little.
- The mind is suspended.
- The movements can last a few minutes or up to twenty or thirty. It is not advisable to continue for longer.
- The movements may stay similar—circular, swaying, bobbing, weaving. They shouldn't become quick or violent. Although that, too, is qi releasing, an environment appropriate to that type of release is essential—a martial arts program, for instance.
- The movements may vary within a session or from session to session. It makes no difference and should be of no concern.
- This is a movement that establishes a return to the most natural of forces, the wise and natural expression of self. This state of awareness is new. You have grounded for earth qi. You have reached to the cosmos

for universal qi. You have brought them both back to your core and allowed them to move through you, connecting your inner and external world.

This is a very important link-up, one that balances, renews, and transforms us and our engagement with life. Take time to integrate what has filled you, changed you, and healed you.

The Eighth Freedom (three to five minutes)

End the movement in the same physical position in which you started:

Relax.

Settle down.

Keep the knees soft.

Sink down in the pelvis.

Elevate the head.

Hold the back relaxed and easily straight.

Breathe to the dan tian.

Relax the arms.

Elbows should be soft and rounded.

Hold the palms facing each other.

This is a time of containment. Feel the skin of your body. Feel the outer membrane of your personal qi field. Feel yourself directly in the center of your

> Instinctive qigong can be done sitting and lying down as well. The process is the same. The movement emanates from the inner feeling to be reflected or exaggerated in the muscles. Then a movement is initiated. This should be an easy, no-stress feeling, a turning within allowing the qi to flow into and through movement.

egg-shaped qi field, contained and tranquil. Your breath is in the dan tian. Now place your palms completely on your abdomen. Feel your qi field center, contents, and boundary. Your body will integrate the changes during this time. Accept whatever change has occurred. Connect through the top of your head to the universe and through the soles of your feet to the Earth. Feel the foundation of Earth completely and fully under you.

Slowly open your eyes, or adjust your vision to be present if your eyes have been open.

This type of qigong, like the others, can be done daily, but not more often

A ll physical conditions evolve in the body from a variety of contributing factors:

Basic genetic health

Trauma reactions

Environmental stresses

Body-nurturing habits

Qigong helps you develop balance, but trusting your own deep wisdom about your pace of integration and awareness is essential. Consciously and unconsciously, you know your own timing. Just keep moving, don't stop or pull away from life.

than that. It is too hard to take in that much qi and then fulfill our obligation to engage with life, "recycling" the qi accumulated. When this gets out of whack, you can have headaches, be irritable, get spaced-out, become an escape artist from life, and fill with unmanifested ideas. Take in what you can work with.

Cautions
If there is discomfort, pain, lightheadedness, loss of balance, nervousness, or aggression, stop the instinctive qigong. Sit down or take a walk, whichever is appropriate, and next time do less, feel less, and take your time.

Mind Regulation and Instinctive Qigong
One strong school of thought believes that the body knows exactly what to do with qi, that it knows where to put it and how to readjust and balance it, that the wisdom of the natural instincts of the body is flawless, and the body only needs the opportunity to do self-healing. According to this school of thought, you would simply rest after doing your instinctive qigong.

Another school of thought adds a helpful suggestion to this idea. If you are aware of ongoing stiffness, a little twinge, or cluttered thoughts that are annoying you, use the qi like a stream of water or air, and just flush them away.

Stiff neck: Breathe into the neck and direct the qi to flow there, exhale, and release it out to the universe.

Headache: Inhale qi into the head, and exhale the ache.

Overly busy thoughts: Inhale qi to the frontal lobe of the brain, and exhale out the thoughts. Sense them tumbling over one another as they pour out.

Lower-back soreness: Inhale qi into the back and abdomen, exhale the pain out the back. Inhale strength into the abdominal muscles.

Eyestrain: Inhale qi into the eyes. Make your vision originate from deep within your head, and exhale out the tension.

Skin problems (any color of skin): Inhale a pink vapor into the skin, hold it there, and then exhale. Repeat until the skin feels tingly.

Nature's wisdom is the route qi naturally follows. Qi is nature's wisdom. The greatest gift qigong can give you is a complete awareness of yourself.

Eventually you will arrive at a point where you can separate the qi from the breath. Then the breathing goes on, slow and natural, to the dan tian, carrying qi with it, and the mind directs more qi directly to where it is needed. Eventually all issues of the body, mind, and spirit are resolved through guiding qi to create personally chosen outcomes. Drawing on qi to create your chosen outcome looks like creating magic, but it isn't magic at all. It is a full and complete understanding of qi, its frequencies, and its management.

This can be a wonderful result of both types of basic qigong expression. And if you long to teach, provide an environment where learners only need to open up to themselves, and self-trust and self-esteem are elevated. This will allow you to become the ultimate teacher, never asking others to leave their own truth to follow you or a system, but instead, to embrace qi to become fully themselves.

questions and answers

What can I realistically expect from qigong?
This is completely dependent on the time you invest in qigong. If you commit to daily practice, you will feel healthier, move more easily, and experience an increasing sense of well-being. If you stay committed, it will change many other aspects of your life for the better.

Where can I get more information on qigong?
Qigong is becoming enormously popular now. As a result, there are many videos, books, Web sites, and classes available. Some excellent books are listed in the Resources section. Look for books that also list resources, to continue to add to your own sources of knowledge.

Should my physician or psychotherapist know I am doing qigong?
Yes. It is good to keep all helping professionals in the loop. And after they witness the benefits forthcoming in you, they may have a better understanding of qigong's ability to help others.

I am movement-impaired. Can qigong benefit me?
Oh yes. Qigong will meet you wherever you are. Some people practice moving only one toe. In these cases, the guiding of qi with the mind makes up a lot of the work.

Will qigong make me look better?
Qigong restores one to better health, and there is nothing that improves looks like improving health. In addition, a daily commitment will produce better skin, restore natural muscle tone, and be generally slimming.

My life has true challenges in it. Can qigong help me?

Qigong will give back more than you invest in it. In this way it is very worth the time, even for those with a challenged life. Once you begin to reap the qigong benefits, you will feel more centered, inwardly nourished, and connected to omnipresence—all good assets to have going for you amidst true challenges.

Will qigong enhance my spiritual development, or will it interfere with my faith, which is not based on Eastern beliefs?

Because qigong connects you to omnipresence, it deeply enhances the feeling of spiritual communion. It is not a faith with guidelines of beliefs and standards. It is a method that enables you to let qi become a more useful resource in every day of your life.

How long does learning qigong take?

Six weeks to three months is the amount of time it takes to settle into sequences of this new form of movement. After that, it is an ever-deepening, open-ended process. Newer students are happy when they have learned it. Masters say they are still learning. That is what makes qigong endlessly interesting.

Are good instructors hard to find?

Instructors are not hard to find. Good instructors are harder to find. Chapter 5 gives you guidelines for choosing. It is also good to remember that the traditional Chinese way—declaring unwavering, lifelong loyalty to one teacher—may not be your way. Qigong was born from the freedom of discovering qi. Don't let all the elaborate qigong systems and vying "masters" take the innocence of it from you.

Is qigong a watered-down t'ai chi or t'ai chi ch'uan?

Actually, qigong predates both by thousands of years. Both t'ai chi ch'uan and t'ai chi probably have their roots in qigong. T'ai chi ch'uan and t'ai chi are more like siblings, children of the same mother. Qigong is the mother.

Will qigong help me with self-esteem issues?

Great question. Qigong leads you back to your own true nature, and despite any fears you may have, your nature is wonderful and uniquely you. As qigong leads you to yourself, your self-acceptance and healthy self-love increase, and then your self-esteem issues dissolve.

Can I do qigong occasionally and get some benefits?

No. In order to know qigong, you must do it.

Will qigong support other forms of exercise?

Yes. You will find that any other sport or fitness activity you enjoy will benefit from qigong. If you feel you have peaked, then add in qigong and see if you don't improve a notch.

Should I teach qigong to others?

Teaching qigong to others often becomes a deep desire because it is so helpful. You may find you want to encourage everyone you know to give it a try. Qigong can produce temporary zealots. Quite quickly, though, it becomes clear that those who will benefit will be drawn to it, and for others, there will be another way.

Sharing the joys of qigong can be done, without taking on too much inappropriate teaching, through "instinctive qigong" (see chapter 19). Qi is everywhere, and the bottom line of qigong is getting qi into the body and then balancing it. It is very possible that our bodies know how to do this intuitively. Trusting this premise, go outside with a friend. Reach up to the sky and inhale, stretch down to or on the earth, and draw in. Then just move exactly as you feel—free, moving, flowing along with life: the movements of freedom. This spontaneous form of qigong is great for you, and wonderful to share with one and all.

Qigong Teachers

Lillibet Gillespie
Travels to teach.
541-890-2497
sifu@itswa-usa.com
www.itswa-usa.com
Shaolin Si Qigong and the Five Elements video
available through Lillibet's Web site.
Order from: www.itswa-usa.com
Or email Lillibet at sifu@itswa-usa.com

To find a qigong teacher:
http://www.qi-energy.com/qigongteachers.htm

Books

Qigong

Chia, Mantak. *Awakening Healing Energy Through the Tao*. Santa Fe, NM: Aurora Press, 1983.

Cohen, Ken. *The Way of Qigong, The Art and Science of Chinese Energy*. New York: Wellspring/Ballantine, 1999.

Diepersloot, Jan: *Warriors of Stillness*, Vol. 1. Walnut Creek, CA: Center for Healing and the Arts, 1995.

Dong, Paul, and Aristide H. Esser. *Chi Gong, The Ancient Chinese Way to Health*. St. Paul, MN: Paragon House, 1990.

Dong, Paul, and Thomas Raffill. *Empty Force: The Ultimate Martial Art*. Boston, MA: Element Books, Inc., 1996.

Frantzis, Bruce Kumar. *Opening the Energy Gates of Your Body*. Berkeley, CA: North Atlantic Books, 1993.

Hong, Liu, and Paul Perry. *The Healing Art of Qigong, Ancient Wisdom from a Modern Master*. New York: Time Warner International, 2000.

Jiao, Guorui. *Qigong Essentials for Health Promotion*. Beijing: China Reconstructs Press, 1988.

Katzman, Shoshanna. *Qigong for Staying Young: A Simple, 20-Minute Workout to Cultivate Your Vital Energy*. New York: Avery of the Penguin Group Inc., 2003.

Lam, Master Kam Chuen. *Chi Kung, The Way of Healing*. London: Gaia Books, 1999.

———. *The Way of Energy*. London: Gaia Books, 1991.

Liang, Shou-Yu, and Wen-Ching Wu. *Qigong Empowerment, A Guide to Medical, Taoist, Buddhist, and Wushu Energy Cultivation*. East Providence, RI: The Way of the Dragon Publishing, 2000.

Lin, Housheng, and Luo Peiyu. *300 Questions on Qigong Exercises*. Guangzhou, China: Guangdong Science and Technology Press, 1994.

Reid, Daniel P. *The Complete Book of Chinese Health and Healing, Guarding the Three Treasures*. Boston, MA: Shambhala, 1994.

———. *A Complete Guide to Chi-Gung*. Boston, MA: Shambhala, 2000.

Shih, T. K. *The Swimming Dragon: A Chinese Way to Fitness, Beautiful Skin, Weight Loss and High Energy*. Barrytown, NY: Station Hill Press, 1989.

Wilson, Stanley D., and Barry Kaplan. *Qigong for Beginners: Eight Easy Movements for Vibrant Health*. NY: Sterling Publishing Co., 1999.

Dr. Yang, Jwing-Ming. *The Essence of Shaolin White Crane: Martial Power and Qigong*. Roslindale, MA: YMAA Publication Center, 2003.

——. *Qigong: The Secret of Youth*. Roslindale, MA: YMAA Publication Center, 2003.

——. *The Roots of Chinese Qigong*. Roslindale, MA: YMAA Publication Center, 1997.

Chinese Medicine

Kaptchuk, Ted K., O.M.D. *The Web That Has No Weaver*. New York: McGraw-Hill/Contemporary Books, 1983, 2000.

Korngold, Efrem, and Harriet Beinfield. *Between Heaven and Earth*. New York: Ballantine Wellspring, 1991.

Ni, Maoshing. *The Yellow Emperor's Classic of Medicine: A New Translation of the Neijing Suwen with Commentary*. Boston: Shambhala, 1995.

Zhen, Li Shi, and G. M. Seifert (ed.). *Pulse Diagnosis*. Brookline, MA: Paradigm Publications, 1985.

Qi and Energy Healing

Eden, Donna, and David Feinstein. *Energy Medicine*. New York: Jeremy Tarcher, 2000.

Jahnke, Roger, O.M.D. *The Healing Promise of Qi*. New York: McGraw-Hill/Contemporary Books, 2002.

Oschman, James. *Energy Medicine: The Scientific Basis of Bioenergy Therapies*. London: Churchill Livingstone, 2000.

Qigong and Massage

Mercati, Maria. *The Handbook of Chinese Massage: Tui Na Techniques to Awaken Body and Mind*. Rochester, VT: Healing Arts Press, 1997.

Reid, Daniel P. *The Tao of Health, Sex and Longevity*. New York: Fireside Book/ Simon and Schuster, 1989.

Dr. Yang, Jwing-Ming and Alan Dougall. *Chinese Qigong Massage*. Roslindale, MA: YMAA Publication Center, 1992.

Nutrition

Pitchford, Paul. *Healing with Whole Foods: Oriental Traditions and Modern Nutrition*. Berkeley, CA: North Atlantic Books, 2002.

Color Healing

Lin, Yun, and Sarah Rossback. *Living Color: Master Lin Yun's Guide to Feng Shui and the Art of Color*. NY: Kodansha America, 1994.

Tappe, Nancy Anne. *Understanding Your Life Through Color*. Carlsbad, CA: Starling Publishers, 1986.

Verner-Bonds, Lilian. *The Complete Book of Color Healing*. Taos, NM: Redwing Book Co., 2000.

Qigong Videos

Cohen, Ken. *Qigong: Traditional Chinese Exercises for Healing Body, Mind and Spirit*. Louisville, CO: Sounds True, Inc., 1996.

Davis, Deborah. *The Spirit of Qigong, Chinese Exercises for Longevity*. Miami, FL: Tapeworm Studio, 1999.

Gillespie, Lillibet. *Shaolin Si Qigong and the Five Elements*. Order from: www. itswa-usa.com.

Katzman, Shoshanna. *Kigong for Staying Young*. New York: Swing Pictures/ Maddog Films, 2003.

Wu, Master Helen, and Master Wen-Ching Wu. *Therapeutic Qigong Video*. East Providence, RI: Way of the Dragon Publishing, 2002.

Related Videos

Cohen, Ken. *Qi Healing, Energy Medicine Techniques to Heal You*. Louisville, CO: Sounds True, Inc., 2002.

Garri, Francesco. *Qigong for Energy*. Broomfield, CO: Gaiam/Living Arts, 1999.

Johnson, Larry, O.M.D. *18 Buddha Hands Qigong, A Qigong Workout*. San Francisco, CA: White Elephant Martial Arts, 1999.

Manning, Laura. *Change the Picture: A Xuan Ming Dao Qigong Video*. Yu-Cheng Huang, 1998.

Dr. Yang, Jwing-Ming. *Chinese Qigong Massage, Self-Massage*. Roslindale, MA: YMAA Publication Center, 1999.

———. Jwing-Ming. *Eight Simple Qigong Exercises for Health*. Roslindale, MA: YMAA Publication Center, 2003.

Audio Cassettes

Cohen, Ken. *Chi Kung Meditations: Taoist Inner Healing Exercises with Ken Cohen*. Louisville, CO: Sounds True, Inc., 1994.

Qigong Associations

Institute of Integral Qigong & Tai Chi
243 Pebble Beach Drive
Goleta, CA 93117 (805-685-4670)
www.feeltheqi.com

International Yan Xin Qigong
Association
P.O. Box 1332
Church Station
New York, NY 10008-1332

info@yanxinqigong.net
www.yanxinqigong.net

China Online
http://chineseculture.about.com/msub_qigong4.htm
Resource for Qigong associations
in China
Worldwide Zhong Yuan Qigong Coordinates
ZY Qigong
626 Malden Ave. East
Seattle, WA 98112
www.zyqigong.org/index.htm

East West Academy of Healing Arts
www.eastwestqi.com
Nonprofit organization in
San Francisco, with programs in many other cities
www.godserver.com
Search engine for qigong and alternative health sites and spirituality sites
World T'ai Chi & QiGong Day
Source for qigong teachers and schools in your area:
http://www.worldtaichiday.org
Links to major associations and publications:
http://www.worldtaichiday.org/Associations.html
Top Qigong Associations at Global Soul Search Directory
http://www.globalsoulsearch.net/alive/Qigong/Associations

Web Sites
www.shaolin.org
www.wahnam.org
www.shaolin-wahnam-center.org
www.jiangtaichi.com
www.peaceabledragon.org
www.ymaapub.com
Go to the search engine Google.com and type in qigong, then settle back for
hours of information.

Chi (qi): The energy pervading the universe and the energy circulating in the human body

Chi kung (qigong): The study of qi

Dan tian: "Field of Elixir," locations in the body that can store and generate qi (elixir) in the body (the lower dan tian is located one and a half inches below the navel, deep in the pelvis)

Di: The Earth

Di qi: Earth qi, the energy of the Earth

Gongfu (kung fu): "Energy-time," all that requires time and energy to learn and accomplish

Houtian qi: Post-birth qi

Huan: Slow

Jing: Essence

Qi: Universal, earthly, and human energy

Ren: Humankind

Ren qi: Human qi

Shen: Spirit

Sifu: Teacher

Taiji: "Grand ultimate"

Taijiquan (t'ai chi ch'uan): Chinese martial art incorporating aspects of qigong

Tian: Heaven or sky

Tian qi: Heaven qi

Wushu: Martial techniques

Xian tian qi: Prebirth qi

Yang: The active, positive, masculine polarity

Yi: Mind

Yin: The passive, negative, feminine polarity

about the author

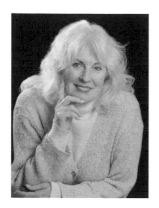

AS A NATIONALLY KNOWN teacher and theorist of the mind/body connection, Ellae Elinwood has drawn upon a background rich in varied experience to conceive her current work. For many years she was an instructor of hatha yoga and t'ai chi, both privately and at colleges, universities, and fitness spas throughout Southern California. She pioneered a program teaching yoga to the elderly in convalescent homes, with remarkable results. She has also been a teacher of shiatsu, "Touch for Health," applied kinesiology, and stress management, and continues as a student of qigong.

A student of psychology, she has trained in the past with body-based therapies, including Bioenergetics and the revolutionary "BodyNamics" works of Lisbeth Marcher.

Through her studies of yoga, Chinese wisdom, and facial exercise, and her investigation into the effects of energy systems and emotions on the face, Ellae developed her book *Timeless Face*, her comprehensive facial toning exercise program (St. Martin's Press).

She has recently had books published on t'ai chi and qigong, *The Everything T'ai Chi and Qigong Book* (Adams Media, 2002) and *Stay Young with T'ai Chi* (Tuttle Publishing, December 2003), as well as numerology, *The Everything Numerology Book* (Adams Media, 2003), and now *Qigong Basics* (Tuttle Publishing, 2004). As an outgrowth of her extensive background, she teaches "Growing Older, Growing Better," a class dedicated to the concept that we are meant to improve as we mature . . . in all ways.

Ellae speaks and gives seminars at universities, colleges, junior colleges, conferences, and massage schools and spas, as well as doing private sessions throughout the United States and Canada.

Ellae now resides with her family in Ashland, Oregon.

Contact Information:

Transformation Through Reflection, Inc.

119 Oak Meadows Place

Ashland, Oregon 97520

Phone: 541-488-4983

E-mail: elinwood@aol.com

Web site: www.ellaeelinwood.com

Lillibet Gillespie

Your teacher for the Shaolin Si sequence in this book, Lillibet Gillespie, has been trained in the Shaolin Si tradition. Lillibet has been teaching t'ai chi ch'uan for twelve years and qigong for seven years. She was born in South Africa and lived most of her adult life in Cape Town, South Africa, where she was introduced to t'ai chi. Her teacher (sifu) was Leslie James Reed of South Africa.

Leslie Sifu was director of the International Taijiquan and Shaolin Wushu Association, headquartered in England. This international association was formed more than three decades ago in Leicester, England, by Association president Derek Frearson Sifu. Today this association is represented in Britain, Scotland, Ireland, Spain, Hungary, Hong Kong, and the United States. The Association is committed to offering traditional and authentic Chinese martial and health arts.

Leslie Sifu studied both major systems (Songshan and Wudangshan) of bio-energetic health attainment and maintenance for more than thirty years. The Songshan heritage was taught by:

- Guo Meng Zhu (sifu) from the Shaolin Monastery, Henan Province, mainland China
- Shi De Tong (sifu and Shaolin monk) from the Shaolin Monastery, Henan Province, mainland China
- Wong Kiew Kit (sifu), Kingdom of Kedah, Malaysia
- Lee Kam Wing (sifu), Hong Kong (Shamsphuipo)

The Wudangshan heritage was taught by:

- Ou Rong Ju (sifu), Fatshan, Guangdong Province, mainland China
- Jiao Hong Bo (sifu), Shaolin Monastery, Henan Province, mainland China
- Wong Kiew Kit (sifu), Kingdom of Kedah, Malaysia

Lillibet Gillespie was privileged to benefit from the richness from Leslie

Sifu's studies and training. She continued to study with Leslie Sifu on a twice-yearly basis after she moved to Ashland, Oregon, in 1997. Presently she is the representative of the International Taijiquan and Shaolin Wushu Association in the United States.

Leslie James Reed passed away unexpectedly on March 3, 2003. Lillibet continues to remain in contact, through training and sharing of information, with instructors of the Association in Cape Town. She endeavors to study with Wong Kiew Kit (Qigong) of Malaysia, who is a fourth-generation successor of Venerable Jiang Nan of the Southern Shaolin Monastery, the recipient of the Qigong Master of the Year award in 1997 in San Francisco and the author of many books. Lillibet also trained with Li Ju Feng from the Philippines in Sheng Zhen Wuji Yuan Gong and with Jiang Jianye of Albany, New York, in the essences of taijiquan and yin/yang medical qigong. She sees herself as an eternal student who endeavors to teach the forms as authentically as possible without losing the essence of this traditional art.

Lillibet is a professional member of the National Qigong Association and continues to read and study to deepen her own practice and expand her knowledge and expertise with special health challenges. She teaches classes in Ashland and Medford, Oregon, specializing in the senior population and in Parkinson's disease, multiple sclerosis, and arthritis. She also teaches private lessons to students with health challenges, such as cancer. Lillibet's teachings include Yang style t'ai chi, Shaolin Hun Yucn Yi qigong, and Shaolin Si qigong. She has been featured in numerous editorials in local newspapers and gives seminars.

ABOUT TUTTLE
"Books to Span the East and West"

Our core mission at Tuttle Publishing is to create books which bring people together one page at a time. Tuttle was founded in 1832 in the small New England town of Rutland, Vermont (USA). Our fundamental values remain as strong today as they were then—to publish best-in-class books informing the English-speaking world about the countries and peoples of Asia. The world has become a smaller place today and Asia's economic, cultural and political influence has expanded, yet the need for meaningful dialogue and information about this diverse region has never been greater. Since 1948, Tuttle has been a leader in publishing books on the cultures, arts, cuisines, languages and literatures of Asia. Our authors and photographers have won numerous awards and Tuttle has published thousands of books on subjects ranging from martial arts to paper crafts. We welcome you to explore the wealth of information available on Asia at **www.tuttlepublishing.com**.